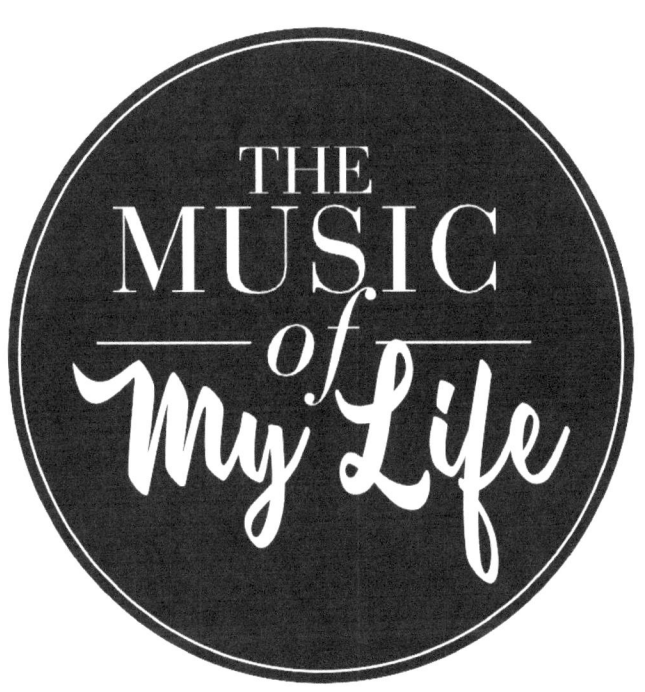

THE MUSIC of My Life

Cleoni Crawford

ROMELO Publications

The Music of My Life

Copyright @ 2019 by Cleoni Crawford
This title is also available as an ebook.
ISBN 978-1-9990430-2-5
Requests for information should be addressed to:

Romelo Publications
406-134 Queen Street East
Brampton, ON
Canada   L6V 1B2

This digital edition: 978-1-9990430-3-2

Romelo Publications 2019

Library and Archives Canada:
Crawford, Cleoni.
The Music of My Life

ISBN 978-1-9990430-2-5

1. Mental Health
2. Christian Life
3. Personal Development

Any information, data, and references are offered as a resource.
They are not intended in any way to be or imply an endorsement
by Romelo Publications.

All rights reserved. No part of this publication may be reproduced,
stored in a retrieval system, or transmitted in any form or by any
means - electronic, mechanical, photocopy, recording, or any other –
except for brief quotations in printed reviews, without the prior
permission of the publisher.

Cover design: Cre8tive Eye Designs
Interior design: Cre8tive Eye Designs
Printed in Canada

*I would like to dedicate this book to my mother Jannett,
sister Feleisha ,dad Clinton, friend Dawn,
my Pastor, Pastor Castro and
APC Ministries who have all been there to support me
despite the difficult times.
Also, I dedicate this book to my son Emmanuel,
mommy loves you with all her heart.
Love you all*

Cleoni.

Table of Contents

vi   Introduction

Chapters

1	1. Big Pharma
11	2. I Made it. But Not Her
19	3. Hidden Opportunities
27	4. From Shame to Praise
33	5. I am Cleoni. I am Bipolar.
47	6. My Saving Grace
57	7. Happy or So I Thought!
73	8. Lean on Me
87	9. Virtual Insanity
101	10. Music Therapy
127	11. Social Media Queen
145	12. Kick Push
155	13. Promiscuous Girl
175	14. Babies are Blessings
187	15. Manic
201	16. Finding Purpose

Introduction

Writing this book was a long time coming. For years, I had been writing bits and pieces of my story in journals and on social media. I knew one day I would write a book.

I had gone through so much and knew that I wanted to encourage someone. I am so glad that I have been able to finally write this story. My aim is to raise awareness for mental health and give you an inside look at what bipolar disorder can look like. In this story, I have been very transparent and have shared as much of my story as I could remember. I have decided to be quite vulnerable and transparent in sharing this story and therefore would like to give a disclaimer as there is one section of the book where I talk about sex. Some people may be uncomfortable with this topic and may want to skip that section of the book. I speak about this in chapter 13. If you would rather skip that part of the book, that's fine.

Sometimes mental illness can be ugly and there are parts of my story that can be troubling. However, if I can help someone to know that they can overcome despite their dark seasons, then I feel like I have accomplished my goal.

For years, I was told I should write a book, but it was only a thought. However, it wasn't until Shelley Jarrett of **SMJ Magazine**, one morning in 2017, asked me to write my story for a future project that we will be working on that I actively started to write this book in 2018. I would go to the library and write and write. Though I was writing, I didn't have a target date. Then, in January 2019, I met my now mentor, Victoria A. Morgan, who challenged me in a mentorship mastermind, to complete my book in one month. I was fearful and did not think it would be possible. However, despite this, I took on the challenge and completed my book in February 2019. I am very thankful that I was able to complete it and hope that you will be inspired.

There are so many people that I would like to thank. First, I would like to thank my family for standing by me in the difficult seasons of my life. I would also like to thank my friends who stood by me. Furthermore, I would like to thank my Pastor, Pastor Castro, and church, APC Ministries for loving me and supporting me despite the difficult seasons I put them through. It has been a rough battle but yet I made it.

Finally, I would like to thank all the people who pre-purchased their copy of my book as this helped me raise the capital to pay for the publishing fees. You are all amazing. I pray that you are all blessed and enlightened by this book and that it teaches you about empathy for those living with mental illness.

The struggle is real y'all.
Blessings, Cleoni.

Chapter 1:
Big Pharma

"Cleoni, go to bed. Why are you staring at me like that?" shouted my mother. And suddenly it happened, my body started to shake wildly until I fell to the ground, continuing to shake. I bit my tongue and blood started to ooze out. Finally, I wet myself. My nightgown was wet and soaked in urine. This was my first epileptic seizure. It was definitely not my last. The next thing I remember was being in the emergency room with wires hooked up to my body as I opened my eyes to see my mother looking over me with concern. She was relieved that I finally regained consciousness. As any mother would be, she was happy that I was all right. Not knowing how I got to the emergency room, I questioned, "where am I and how did I get here?" My mother then explained that I had my first epileptic seizure. I was only 12 years old at the time and did not understand epilepsy. However, epilepsy would soon become a part of my life. I remember going to my first neurologist, where they told my mother that I would have epilepsy for a long time, maybe even the rest of my life. I became sorrowful. However, they also gave me my first medication.

That was the beginning of 'Big Pharma' being introduced into my life. I would take the medication but I would still have seizures. It was like a routine. Every Saturday night, I would watch Mad TV with my younger brother and then fall asleep on the couch. When my mother came in from a show or a party, she would find me on the sofa and ushered me to my bed, and then it would happen, I would have a seizure. It was either at the top of the stairs, in the bathroom, or as I was about to climb into my bed. No matter how it happened it would happen. We kept trying different medication and nothing worked until I tried Epival. This medication worked very well. It reduced my seizures drastically from weekly to quarterly. However, it made me gain a lot of weight and I was overly tired. After years of dealing with epilepsy, we as a family learned that if I was sleeping not to wake me as this might trigger a seizure. With that said, if my family found me sleeping, they all knew never to wake me in fear that I might become ill and have a seizure. Having epilepsy became very difficult. I would seize at school, parties and out in the street. Hospitals became my new best friend. Despite taking medication, I would still have seizures. Then I met a new neurologist, Dr. Yufe. I really liked him. Due to my complaints about excessive weight gain and tiredness, he changed my medication and put me on something new called Lamictal also known as Lamotrigine. This medication worked very well. With that said, I still had to ensure that I got enough sleep because not getting enough would trigger a seizure. Throughout high school, my seizures seemed to be under control. I did not have as many seizures as I did in the past. I was grateful.

Entering high school, West Humber Collegiate Institute was awesome. I made some great friends and I enjoyed my time there. I was smart and got good grades. I was an A student. Though, an A student, I loved to party. At the tender age of 13, I started to go clubbing with my adopted sister. I was only 13 but I had the body of an 18 year old. I looked good. I would dance all night, as I loved music.

When I was 16, I met a biracial man, a mixture of Chinese and black. Like most men, he wanted sex. We dated and I lost my virginity at 16. Sweet sixteen. That's when it started. Over the next five years I had multiple partners. They were different races and different religions. My relationships were usually short lived. However, I did have a main partner over that time; he was my default partner. I really enjoyed having sex with him. We never really dated but he did take me to my prom. Later on in life, I would discover why I enjoyed sex so much.

During the time I was growing up, it was customary for us to relocate on a regular basis. Almost every time we moved, I had to change schools. By the time I was in my mid-teens, I had been to seven schools. This one time we moved to Bathurst and Wilson. I loved this place. Though much smaller than our big house in Etobicoke, it was on top of a store and the neighbourhood was quiet and peaceful

While living in Bathurst and Wilson, I had to change schools again. I went to Sir Sandford Fleming Academy for one year for grade 10. The friends I made were mostly men. I really didn't like my school and wished I would I go back to West Humber. For the first time ever, I got into a fight and lost. I was beaten up by a white girl. It was very shameful. People made fun of me and I grew tired of that school.

So, the following year in grade 11, I went back to West Humber. Every day I would take the bus for 1 hour just to be at a school where my friends were. I was happy again.

I stayed at West Humber until the end of grade 12 and loved it. While I was there, I started to go to church at 16 with my best friend Genice. I would take the bus to her house Sundays and get picked up by the church, NLPC. I really liked that church. It was different.

I still went to parties but I was changing. Sunday school, led by the Pastor's son Brother Richard, was challenging my beliefs. I started to tell Brother Richard, who was the youth pastor that I would get baptized soon but would keep changing my mind. One day at 17 while in grade 12 I decided to get baptized. It felt so refreshing. However, when I went home I was mocked by my family and called "Gre-tian" short for a fake Christian. They didn't believe that I could be a Christian because of my partying ways. However, twenty years later this Christian is still here.

Also at 17, I was forced to leave my mother's home due to stress and the increase in seizures. My brother had started stealing from me, such as my clothing, money, or whatever he could find. This caused us to get into fist fights. I would threaten him to hurt him with a knife. Then I would have a seizure due to the stress. It became very serious.

To escape this, I moved into my paternal grandmother's home. It was very different. My grandmother was a disciplinarian. She was strict and didn't speak my love language. According to Gary Chapman's book, **The Five Love Languages**, my love language was affirmation. When I lived with my mother, she would constantly affirm me through praises. She would remind me that I could do and be anything. She would tell me that I was smart and it gave me strength. I didn't realize how powerful words could be at the time, but that was what kept me together. My grandmother's love language was giving gifts, which she showed me daily by providing a clean, stable home with a home cooked meal.

This was good for me. I needed stability and she provided that. However, she never affirmed me. Sometimes, she would say things like, *"you're not smart enough"* or *"you should stay on welfare and forget university."* This hurt a lot. However, I had the years of affirmations from my mother to lean on. This kept me going.

Months later, after applying to 3 universities, I finally got the acceptance package from the University of Toronto. I was ecstatic. This was the best news I could ever get; this was proof that I was smart. It made me feel so good. However, one day, my best friend and church brother, Robert came over. While we were joking around, my grandmother berated me and cussed me and called me nasty. This was it. I had already started to become depressed with my grandmother's comments. My best friend was in the living room. While there, saddened and angry with tears streaming down my face, I picked up a knife and put it to my throat. I was going to kill myself until my friend came into the room and shouted, *"Cleoni, no!"* He grabbed the knife away from me and comforted me while I sobbed. Sadly, those words were starting to affect my mental health.

When university came, I was a Christian and therefore had conservative beliefs. I started to wear skirts all the time and stopped partying. With all the parties happening, it became very difficult. I started to feel like I didn't fit in. Though I made friends, I didn't have a social life with them. I focused on my friends from church.

University was hard. I took Psychology, Sociology, French and Spanish. Although they were very interesting, I started to fall behind. For the first time in my life, I got C's and failed a course. This was so discouraging. I was put on academic probation. If I did not increase my grades, I would be suspended for one year. Sadly, at the end of my second year, I didn't increase my grades and was suspended for a year. This was devastating.

In addition to this, my epilepsy came back due to lack of sleep. I would have various seizures on campus and in class. This was so embarrassing. I was taken to various downtown hospitals. It was so bad that I wound up being admitted to every hospital downtown from Mount Zion to Toronto General. To add insult, I would have seizures at home. I would go into the bathroom in my slip and would fall off the toilet with my underwear down. This became a problem because my grandmother's tenants would find me. My grandmother would cuss me off for not dressing modest enough at bed. To prevent being exposed, my grandmother bought me more modest nightgowns. Though one problem was solved as I was covered up, this did not stop the seizures.

While suspended, I applied for numerous jobs and finally got hired by Bell Mobility call centre. I worked at Bell Mobility for 2 years. After my first year, I decided to go back to school to complete my degree. I worked on the student schedule for a year and then quit the job because it was becoming too difficult to manage the two. I returned back to school and changed my program. I started to take Commerce courses like Economics, Accounting and Calculus. I didn't do too well in these courses. So, I came back the following year and changed to focus on Spanish and History. My grades improved drastically as I started to get As and Bs again. I was so proud of myself.

However, due to my GPA being low from my Commerce courses, I was put on academic probation and was up for suspension again. This suspension was far more serious: it was supposed to be for three years. And I only had two credits left to graduate. I begged and appealed the decision and praise God, they showed me mercy. They let me complete my year.

This was 2005. Here I was, living again with my mother at a new address close to Jane and Sheppard. My sisters would have friends come over all hours of the night which made it difficult for me to study. It was imperative that I did well in school especially since it was my last year. I decided to move out and live on campus. I found a cheap dorm for only $550 per month called Tartu College. It was tiny and I shared the apartment with 4 roommates. One of my roommates was a graduate student but had the worst body odour ever known to man. I think she was a partially homeless. I don't know. While on campus, I started to make new friends and got invited to a few parties. It was a nice change. However, I declined the invitations to go out because I was a Christian whose beliefs didn't support the lifestyle of clubbing.

In my last year, I took two African History courses. These courses and the respective instructors changed my life. My two teachers were phenomenal and got me to change how I viewed black women in society. Afua Cooper taught me about African Canadian History and Nakanyike Musisi taught me about Elite Black Women. These courses were powerful as they inspired me. I decided to create a non-profit organization called Black S.E.E.D. I do not remember what the acronyms stood for but I do remember the impact it had on my life. I became very obsessed with this new organization that I was forming. I was going to register it as a non-profit and bring in mentors and professionals into at-risk communities like Jamestown in Rexdale and inspire the black community into pursuing entrepreneurship.

I spent all my time on this new organization but then something happened. I had a shift in my behavior. This was the first occurrence in what has become a lifelong cyclical pattern.

I started to stay up really late at night and travel at night because I thought I was a spy. I thought that I was on a mission to help black people. I had the answers. I tried to recruit my friends from church and didn't get much response. I felt rejected but yet I continued to work on Black S.E.E.D. I spent hundreds of dollars on supplies for my new organization. I would travel all around the city at 2-4 in the morning.

Other people started to notice my behaviour and grew concerned. However, no one had the courage to tell me that something was wrong. One day, I went to my pastor to tell him about my idea and he discouraged me from doing it. But in my eyes, he didn't know what he was talking about, so I ignored him. I grew worse. I started to talk very fast and ramble from subject to subject.

January 2006 came and my OSAP check arrived. I spent almost all of my living expenses money on more supplies for the organization. I remember taking these supplies to my grandmother's house. She knew that something was wrong, but instead of talking with me she cussed me out. She said, *"You need to stop this crap and relax yourself. You are going from here to there and you are not making any sense."* I ignored her efforts and went back to peace and privacy of my dorm.

My grandmother's words were a premonition that the 'up' period of this cyclical pattern was to be followed by a 'down' period. One morning that January, I tried to get up out of bed and I just couldn't. I started to cry uncontrollably. I didn't eat and I stayed in my room. I cried a lot and didn't want to go to class or go for my morning jog as I had started training for a marathon with a group called Jeans Marines. I lost all desire to do anything. When I finally left my apartment, I put no effort into finding something to wear and wore my house clothes. I would roam the streets and would cry for no apparent reason. I would also go to subway platforms and try to talk myself into jumping off the platform, convincing myself that it would ease the pain. Though the thoughts were there, I couldn't follow through.

I decided that it was time I got help. I called my best friend Genice and told her that I needed help. I do not know who suggested CAMH but that is where we went. She stayed with me and comforted me. That was the first day I learned the term Bipolar II. When I explained my behaviour over the past two months, they had told me that I am exhibiting signs that I had Bipolar II. According to the DSM 5, there are two types of Bipolar Disorder: Bipolar I, which has highs and lows with mania and Bipolar II, which has highs and lows with hypomania. Hypomania is when you are extremely energetic, talkative, and confident with many creative ideas.

Based on the diagnosis, I was told that my disorder was not too bad and I didn't need medication. I was referred to see a school psychiatrist. I would go weekly to see the psychiatrist and she was very helpful. While doing this, I would also continue jogging again every Saturday with my group the Jeans Marines. I also returned back to school. The feelings of depression decreased and my energy was starting to come back.

Then one day on Monday March 27th, 2006, I learned that my cousin, Jermaine Brown, was just murdered. He was 22 years old and had a son. It was heartbreaking for me. I remember being in class and breaking down after seeing a newspaper reminding me of his death. My teacher consoled me. It was helpful but this was truly difficult for me. I went to the funeral and sobbed at his passing. He was far too young to die. This was hard.

Because of this added stress, I stayed in counselling for 6 months, I was discharged from seeing my psychiatrist and was finally doing better. I had found out something about myself that wasn't just epilepsy, and was going to be part of my life from now on. Still, it would be another 6 years before I would encounter another bipolar episode.

Chapter 2:
I Made It...But Not Her!

I finally finished my last credits and was ecstatic. I was going to graduate. It was really going to happen. I took my graduation photos and felt very proud. Another accomplishment at the time was my training. I had spent 8 months training for a marathon in Columbus, Ohio. I did a 5km and 10km run in Toronto, but it was now time for the big event. In October 2006, I completed my first 42 km full marathon. It took me 5.5 hours to complete the race. I felt so accomplished. It took me a while to complete it, but I did it. Then, the following month came, November 2006. It was my graduation. I was so excited. I started to think back. After all the years of getting sick, being suspended, the death of my cousin and then being diagnosed as Bipolar, I was grateful.

I remember standing in the line waiting for my name to be called. I was shaking as I thought back on what it took for me to get to this place. Then, finally, I heard my name. As I took my diploma and shook the teacher's hand, here it goes, I shouted out a loud, "Hallelujah." People started to laugh and clap as I walked off the stage. I can and can't believe I just did that, but I was overjoyed. It was only God that caused me to graduate despite my trials. At my graduation, I was only allowed two people. Since my father wasn't in town, I invited my mother and my Pastor. They were both very proud of me. I did it.

Just before graduation, I obtained a job at a law firm as a secretary through an employment agency. I did so well that the company offered a salary and hired me. I loved my job and the atmosphere of a law office. Though I worked as a secretary, my goal was to one day become a lawyer. While working, I completed my LSAT and didn't get the grades I hoped for. In addition, after seeing the amount of hours that the lawyers had to put in, I decided that I no longer wanted to be a lawyer. Soon after, I had another career goal.

One night, very early in the morning, I woke up and came up with the idea to design skirts and create an online directory that connected businesses online. I wrote my business plan that morning and shared my idea with my bosses. They thought it was great. That is why it came as a great shock that seemingly without warning, a few weeks later, I was fired from my job in April 2007 due to my lateness.

However, God knew what he was doing. One day, while in the JVS Employment Centre in Jane-Finch mall looking for a new job, I learned about a program called Summer Company. Summer Company was a government-sponsored program that provided $3000 to students who wanted to start their own business. I was taken aback with surprise as I already had a business plan and idea ready. The application was due in 2 weeks and I arrived just in time. I completed the paperwork and was accepted for the program. I started my new business in May 2007 and was so excited. I was doing something new and exciting. I was going to sell my skirts in my new company C-virtue. I designed a website and within one month, I received 400 views. I was excited.

Then another tragic event happened. On Saturday June 2, 2007 at 9am, I was awoken to a scream. My mother screamed my name and I ran upstairs.

She was breathing heavily and could barely speak. *"There was a car accident, one dead, one alive. It's Aleisha and Monique."*

Aleisha was my sister and Monique was her best friend who was living with us. My mother temporarily and unofficially adopted her, her sister, Chanel and brothers Trevon and Andrew. They were family. My heart sank and started to beat heavily. She continued, *"The police are on the way to explain everything, call Feleisha and Clinroy"* (my sister and brother).

I started to make calls and we gathered in our living room. Both of our families waited on the police. The police finally arrived and told us the details. Apparently, my sister, Aleisha and her best friend was also like a sister, Monique were in a tragic car accident. They were in a taxi on their way from their aunt's house and were T-boned by a young man, Chevon Joseph, 15, who was being chased by police as he had stolen his mother's car. As the police continued to tell the story, my sister, Feleisha, screamed, got up, and ran outside crying hysterically. She could not believe it. Our sister. This couldn't be real. They continued to say that we needed to go to the hospital and identify the body of the living teen. The living teen was at Sunnybrook Hospital. The police left. Then, suddenly, Chanel, Monique's sister arrives at the house. We tell her the story and she runs outside holding her head screaming and crying. My sister was crying but went after her. We then got in our cars and rushed to the hospital.

When we arrived at the hospital, we were all frantic and on pins and needles. We did not know which sister was in the waiting room. Was it Aleisha? Was it Monique? Then the doctor came out and spoke to my mom and Judith (the mother of Monique) and said they could both come in and identify the living daughter. When they returned, it turns out that the living daughter was my sister. She was on life support. Monique was dead. Her body parts lay splattered over the ground at the intersection of Islington Avenue and Finch

Avenue West. When we learned the truth, we were both sad and relieved. One of them was living. However, one of them had died. I stood watching Judith, Chanel, Trevon and Andrew sob as the reality of their sister and daughter was dead. It was surreal. I was grateful that my sister was still living. Well, at least we still have one of them living, but she was in grave condition. As the hours passed, more and more people came to the hospital. My aunt, cousins, and her father gathered at the hospital. We waited for a miracle. I called up my friends and church family asking for prayer.

The following day, I went to my church begging them to pray for my sister as she lay on life support. I wanted them to come to the hospital to pray for her. I wanted them to pray for a miracle at the hospital. None of them came. I went back to the hospital and the doctors gather us together and said we needed to make a decision. He declared her brain dead and wanted us to donate her organs before they could no longer be used. He wanted to know if we wanted to take her off life support. It had only been a day. I wanted to wait a bit longer. My mother decided to take her off of life support. I was so angry and resentful. How could she do this? They then left the hospital while I remained. I decided that I would stay and pray for a miracle until they disconnected my sister. I truly believed that if I prayed hard enough that God could cause her to rise up into consciousness. I prayed all night and did not sleep. Finally I stopped praying for her to rise up. I said, *"Lord, if you choose to let her die, you have to pay me back."* He chose to let her die. At 8am on Monday June 4th, 2007, I watched as they wheeled my sister out of ICU into the operating room. I was devastated.

I came home to a house filled with people. There were all kinds of people dropping in offering their help and condolences. This lasted for days until the funeral. The phone rang non-stop. Finally, I decided to create a Facebook group that had the information about the funeral and changed our voicemail to reflect this. This was so helpful to many people. The funeral was held at Faith Sanctuary with over 1100 people and the media in attendance. Since the two girls were so close, we decided to bury them together. They were "two peas in a pod." The coffins lay side-by-side at the altar. However, Monique's casket remained closed due to the nature of her death. I remember walking up the aisle to take a final look at my sister. She was so cold but her makeup was done nice. She wore a beautiful gown with jewellery. However, her body looked stuffed. There were all kinds of people there. There were friends, family, and classmates and well-wishers. Throughout this whole time, I had kept it together. I consoled everyone because I was the Christian in the family. I was the one that everyone expected to keep it together. However, finally, at the graveyard, I no longer could hold it together. I started to wail and scream. I fell to my knees and screamed my sister's name as they lowered my sister and Monique's coffins. As soon as I screamed, the rest of my family started to wail. My brother fell to the ground crying. It was horrible.

While all of this was happening, my team with Summer Company was so supportive. They gave me permission to leave the program if I needed to grieve. I chose to continue running my business. It was hard but I did it. During that same summer, once the funeral ended, I told my mother that I would be leaving. Everyone had leaned on me for far too long. I needed a break. I decided to go to New York to stay with my aunt. I watched The Color Purple with Fantasia and met Tyler Perry. Then I took the bus to Atlanta, Georgia. I had been reading about Martin Luther King Jr. and wanted to visit his memorial grounds. Then, I went to visit the church of a powerful preacher I met in Canada. It was a great healing vacation. When I returned, I continued with the program and successfully finished it. At the end, I decided that I would return back to school to study fashion. I wanted to expand my business. I registered for school and would start in January 2008. So I had a few months to wait.

While waiting, I went to the Bereaved Families of Ontario to grieve. I would attend their support groups and listen to other grieving siblings talk about their family members. It was difficult but I became better. I decided that I would work with the Bereaved Families of Ontario to create a support group. Then I took scholarship in memory of my sister and Monique's name. I held a press conference at the Queen's Park Legislative Media Room to promote this. I was featured all over the media for this program. Some thought it was good and there were others that doubted that this would last. Due to my work, I had received an award for Outstanding Youth Award by JVS Strictly Business event. Then, I hosted an event called *Gospel, Arts N Praize* in memory of my sister, Aleisha and Monique. I raised $1500 from this event and was so proud of myself. It was hosted on June 2008.

In January 2008, I started school at George Brown College in the Fashion Design and Techniques program. I was doing really well and got good grades in the first semester. I even had the opportunity to meet a mentor, Shernett Swaby of Project Runway Canada. The second semester began. I did well until there was an incident. A friend of mine started to bully my other friend and I decided to step in. She told me to mind my business. I told her to stop messing with someone who could not defend themselves. She decided to curse me out. I responded and retaliated cursing her back. This continued throughout the hallways and down the stairs into the cafeteria. I had my toolbox. She continued to taunt me. Finally, I went into my toolbox and pulled out my scissors. I pointed them at her and she responded, *"What are you gonna do cut me?"* I realized what I did and put the scissors back and knocked her out. She scratched me and we were on top of each other. Then, suddenly two security officers came and broke us apart. She screamed, *"Charge her, she tried to cut me."* The police were called and for the first time in my life, I was arrested. I went to jail and they put me in a questioning room. After a few hours, they finally, released me on my own recognizance. However, I would have to come to court.

I returned back to school. It was not the same. I was given a restraining order and was not permitted to be within 100 metres of the victim; this created problems. If I saw her on campus, I was supposed to go the other way. Also, if we had classes together, I could not be in that class with her. It wasn't fair. I tried to work with my teachers but in the end of the day, it was decided that I would be suspended for a year. I was required to have a psychiatric assessment to return.

Chapter 3:
Hidden Opportunities

Since I loved fashion, I decided to ask if I could intern with Shernett Swaby and she agreed. She was fabulous and I learned a lot. Her work was so detailed and she was a phenomenal fashion designer. Finally, in 2009, after being with her for 7 months, I decided to create my own collection of modest clothing. She helped me with the patterns and some of the sewing. I hosted my first fashion show. I did a lot of work and got my city counsellor to sponsor the cost of the event. He became the keynote speaker. Also, I designed a suit for Judy Sgro, Member of Parliament for the former York West ward. The fashion show was held at the Yorkwoods Public Library Theatre. It was covered by the media and was a packed house. I was so proud of myself.

A few months later, I was asked to appear on 100 Huntley Street, the Full Circle edition. They wanted to learn about my new clothing collection of modest clothing for women and to share my story about depression. It was a really great interview. It aired on Global TV, Crossroads TV and was uploaded on YouTube. Since then, I was featured on CTV, Rogers TV, the Globe and Mail and Toronto Life. I hosted two more fashion shows since then. I was getting a lot of media attention for my business but was not making enough sales. That was frustrating.

I decided to get a job to be able to fund my dream. The Ontario Public Service hired me as a temporary employee through an employment agency. After two months of working there, I got offered a contract to work directly for the Ontario Public Service. While there, I decided to get a new office for my business in Downsview Park. The rent was cheap and I was slowly getting my name out again. This time, I decided to focus on making skirts rather than full outfits. I decided to have a fashion show at the Clothing Show 2010. It was a great opportunity. I would work my full time job and then come to my office at nights and on the weekends. It was difficult but I did it for months.

 I really enjoyed my job and requested to do a job shadow with the Executive Assistant. Due to office politics and one jealous co-worker who was ahead of me, my boss did not approve the job shadow. However, they kept telling me how exceptional I was. I was disappointed. I continued working but this disappointment started to affect me.

 My epilepsy returned and I started to come in late for work because of that. I decided to tell my employers about my condition and was doubted. They questioned why I did not tell them before. I told them I didn't have to tell them about my condition. They then gave me this questionnaire that would prove that I was incompetent of working my job. When I showed it to my doctor, he recommended that I not fill it out. I decided to show it to my union rep and they said half of the questions written were illegal. From that point on, I decided to get my union involved. I was then given a letter of termination. I would read through the laws regarding my situation and found out that they could not just fire me like that but had to give me 16 weeks' pay or keep me employed for 16 weeks. They decided to pay me out. I was given $10,000 to leave. My last day was July 29, 2011. Since I was laid off, I qualified for Employment Insurance. I took this to mean that God was giving me a chance to focus on my business. So that is what I did.

In May 2011, our landlord decided to sell the house and we were to move. I found a place for myself in a basement close to Jane and Finch. I loved it. The rent was reasonable at $600 per month. It was going well until one day in mid-August it started to rain. It rained so bad, that it created a flood in my apartment. The water kept rising and rising and more of my furniture got damaged. My sofa, cabinets, dressers, drawers and more were flooded. I called my landlord to help me get rid of the water. He helped but it was too late. All my furniture was damaged. I decided to check the drawers and then I found it; it was mold. Mold was growing all over my apartment. Not only were my furniture water damaged but they were also filled with mold. I decided to move out immediately because of what I learned about mold. I asked for my money back for August and was given it back.

I called my mother for help but I could not live with her. She recommended I contact my maternal grandmother, Kacheta. I contacted her and was allowed to move into her place. With all my furniture destroyed, I moved with only clothing and a few totes with my fashion stuff. It was hard because it was a condo and I was living in a room as opposed to an apartment. I had not lived in a room in a long time. It was a hard transition.

Two weeks later, my church went on a trip to Atlanta, Georgia to go to the Singles Conference hosted by my favourite preacher. It was such a powerful trip. I learned so much about myself. I came back with a revelation that God would use my social media to reach the masses and that I needed to resign from the Youth Committee and Choir from my church. These two ministries were causing me stress and it was time to leave them. I came back and wrote my resignation and started to be treated badly by my church. That was just the beginning.

A month later, I received an eviction notice from my landlord for my office at Downsview Park. This caught me by surprise as I just moved into the building. I had just started decorating and buying supplies. I was devastated. I had six months to find a new place or get rid of my equipment. So I decided to take a trip to Chicago and then Atlanta. I went to visit my mentor Shernett Swaby in Chicago. She had moved there for business, as she no longer felt that Toronto was good for high fashion. I visited her and had a great time. From Chicago, I took the bus to Atlanta. I felt so refreshed in Atlanta. I spent my time with my new friends from the DeKalb United Pentecostal Church and had a blast. While there, I started to develop feelings for a gentleman down in Atlanta. Sadly, he was not interested in me like that. I came back to Toronto, feeling good about myself but stressed about my office.

Due to the revelation I had received about social media being the place that I would have my greatest impact, I started to make daily videos. These videos were about random topics but tied to an inspirational message at the end. I started to get various followers and met many people online. However, my church started to become very critical about my videos. They didn't like them. They started to call me crazy. Some thought my videos and posts were cool, others thought I was spending too much time on it. I started to spend more and more time on Facebook and YouTube and loved it.

However, suddenly things changed. In January of 2012, I made a video called Breach of Contract against my former employers. I said they had breached their contract against me and fired me for unjust reasons. I posted this video everywhere and to all the employees. I started to write threatening letters to my employer because I was angry that I lost my job. I called them various types of profane names until I got a letter from the legal counsel at the Ontario Public Service asking me to cease and desist. During this time, my church started to change how they treated me. They started to call me crazy and started to avoid being around me. This made me angrier.

The day came when I had to move out of my office. Sadly, rather than put all my equipment in storage, I decided to sell all three of my industrial sewing machines, rolling racks, and tables. I was devastated that I was losing my place. But I moved out and that was the end of that.

However, months later, I was given two opportunities. I saw it as God opening doors for me. In Atlanta, my friend's mother had a small store in the flea market and was thinking of selling my goods. She made it sound like it was a good place to sell my goods. So, I decided to go down to Atlanta in May 2012 to see the place and try and sell a few skirts. She sold one skirt. I was very disappointed and decided not to continue to sell my skirts there. I decided to give away many of my skirts to the ladies in Atlanta.

When I returned, the second opportunity I was given was to sell my clothing in a retail store that would be a collective. I got accepted into the program and got to the sell my clothing in this new store called Ascend. Ascend was located 5 minutes from my former church. However, NOT one person, from the church I had attended since I was 16, visited my new store. I was so hurt. I couldn't believe it. However, right around that same time, my current church, Apostolic Pentecostal Church of Pickering, contacted me to do an interview with me about Excellence. They saw my work and wanted to interview me about my business.

While my previous church was shunning me and treating me badly, this new church was accepting me. One day I decided to go to church after sending a mass text saying that I would be going to church and saying nothing and waiting for God to intervene. I walked all the way from my apartment to Islington and then jumped on the bus to church while wearing my new red gown. When I got to church, I was blocked from going in. I was told that I was going to create a scene and they were not letting me in. I started to curse and swear and reminded them that my stepmother was there and was expecting me. They didn't care. They said they would call the police and I threw them my phone and said to call them. Then the Pastor came out and said that he was sick of my nonsense and asked me to leave his church and never return back. I called my father and he picked my stepmother and I up and we left. I went home both relieved and sad. For months, my friends told me to leave my church and find a new one but I just couldn't. I was praying that God would turn things around. He never did.

When my Pastor kicked me out of my church, I was confused. I did not know where else to go. All the churches that were in my organization were under his supervision. There were 25 churches that were under his supervision and I knew that if I went to one of the churches, I would not get a fair chance. With that said, I stayed at home and had church in my bedroom with Bishop TD Jakes' E-church for 8 weeks. This was the longest that I had stopped attending church.

It was Wednesday June 27th when I got the call that my aunt was in the hospital. I rushed to the hospital, as this was my favourite aunt; her name was Urande Dornevil. She had two adult children and was only 44 years old. Apparently, she had overdosed on drugs and was now in a coma. Full of zeal, I cursed the devil and claimed that this was a just a test of our faith. I spoke to my stepmother; Emlin aka Fine and we started to pray. We went to the chapel and started to call on God for healing. I took of my video and started to film myself praying for my aunt. I truly believed that my God was going to deliver her. However, on Sunday July 1, 2012, my precious aunt was taken off of life support. I was devastated. She was gone.

The following day, due to my Facebook activity and video blogs, my mother decided to come to my house to speak to me. She demanded that I admit myself into the hospital. She said that she couldn't be silent any longer. Around that time, I started to discover the character Jezebel and started to call my mother Jezebel. I felt as though she wanted to hurt me. So, I called my father and stepmother and friend. My father was pissed. He rebuked her. After talking it out, we decided we would call the ambulance to check me out. Then we called 911. The paramedics convinced me to go to the hospital.

I thought everything was going well and then, it happened, I was given a Form 1 and required to stay in the hospital for 3 days. I was upset and pissed that I had ever listened to the ambulance staff. I was sent to the William Osler Hospital for 3 days. I paced the hallways back and forth. I would look out the window longing for my freedom. This was the first time that I was put back in the hospital ever since 2006 for mental health.

I couldn't believe that the doctors did not believe me. I told myself I was fine. So, I started to compile a list of people to contact. I frantically called all my friends, family and church family for help. A few people visited but no one could help. I was livid with my mother who I had now called Jezebel. I blamed her. She was the reason why I was locked up. As far as I was concerned, she was unsaved and therefore, needed to repent and get the spirit of discernment. In my eyes, she was sinning against God by having me put in the hospital. I blamed the spirit of Jezebel for its role in my family. I called myself a Prophetess and was convinced that Jezebel wanted to destroy me. She wanted to create division in my family and pit mother against daughter. I started to cuss Jezebel with Jamaican profanity in my journal.

Considering that there was nothing to do, I spent a lot of time journaling. I wrote a letter to the psychiatrist that was seeing me, Dr. Pat. I claimed that he and the staff were treating me like a nigger. I was angry. All I wanted to do was make a difference through my business and did not understand why so many people were trying to stop me. I wrote that I had forgiven him and wanted to be released. As far as I was concerned, I was not a danger to others or myself and therefore should be released. At that point, in my head, I was not bipolar but merely under stress from the way my church was treating me. I just wanted to go home so I could grieve the passing of my beloved aunt.

It was very difficult being in the mental hospital. I would watch people walk pass me as though they were zombies. They had no life in them. They dragged their feet and slowly moved through the halls. According to me, I did not belong. I was different then these people. "I was not crazy. I did not lose my mind," I told myself. I woke up Wednesday morning and started to journal. I first noticed the time. It was 7:35 am. I started to recount my past few days and started to write about it. Then, I started to create my first sermon because in my mind, I was going to preach a sermon one day. I continued to write my sermon entitled, "And it was good." After writing this, I started to write that I needed a lawyer. I wanted to sue the hospital for defamation of character for discrimination. I wanted a black civil rights lawyer to help me. My plan was to find one when I left the hospital.

Chapter 4:
From Shame to Praise

It was Thursday July 5th, 2012 and once again I woke up early. I had slept for 10 hours because of the sleeping pills that I was forced to take. I tried to refuse medication but apparently my parents told the doctors to force me to take the pills. I felt like the hospital had treated me like a dog and nigger. I was not a nigger; I was a Child of God. They had made a mistake, I claimed. They had put a millstone around their neck and were going down I said. God would judge the hospital for their ill treatment of me. They forced me to take a needle in my butt and sleeping pills. I was saddened that my parents chose to listen to the doctor rather than their own child. During my stay the hospital nurse gave me two options; 1) take the sleeping pills freely or 2) get strapped down to my bed and be forced to take it. I was upset because I felt like I lost all rights.

This was my release date. I woke up so weak and tired due to the sleeping pills they gave me. At 12 pm they discharged me after it was determined that I was fine. However, I was so tired. I arrived home just before 1pm. I slept till 11:35pm then went back to sleep till 7:00 am. Though I slept almost 18 hours, I still felt sluggish. My aunt arrived and I was so hungry but couldn't keep my eyes open. I had to beg my aunt to feed me. This was ridiculous. I was definitely going to sue the doctor for their treatment.

Saturday July 14, 2012 was exactly one month since my store opened and also was the day of my aunt's funeral. It was held at the Prayer Palace. The funeral had many people. I spent most of the time comforting my cousins as they had lost their mother. They were heartbroken. However, at the reception, the mood was light and fun. By the end of the day, there was music, fun, food and dancing. Despite her death, I felt that God was going to turn things around for my family.

In August I went to my current church, Apostolic Pentecostal Church of Pickering (APC) for the REAP Conference. I hadn't been in a church in 8 weeks. Like I mentioned earlier, that was the longest I had ever been away from church. This church was packed and full of energy. The Holy Ghost was moving. People were clapping, dancing, jumping and shouting. It was on fire. I went there over four straight days and it was amazing. Though I loved this church, I truly felt that my next church would be in Stone Mountain, Georgia. I felt like that was my true home as I was done with Canada. Canada had taken too much from me and I wanted a new start. So, after the conference, I stayed at APC for 2 weeks and then went to Georgia.

While in Georgia, I went to the Singles Conference and was truly blessed. The speakers all spoke about *"deadly wounds"* and how it can affect someone. It was almost as if God was letting the church recognize that not everything that was happening to me was my fault but could actually be from God. After the service, I went to fellowship with the members of the DUPC (DeKalb United Pentecostal Church) family and it was great. Later that night, since I didn't have a place to stay, I decided to take Miss Sadie's friend's number, Darlene, as she had a room for rent. I stayed at her house for one night, pay her rent but didn't get the key or the receipt.

I wish I had insisted on it.

The following morning, I get picked up by Dorrell (a church brother) and we go to church. It was such a blessing. After the service Joseph (another church brother) took me out for a drive to the beach. The water was dirty but we had fun nonetheless. The only problem was we had the landlord's key. When we got back to the house, Darlene was so upset because she was worried about her key. Finally, she calmed down. My friends, Dorrell and Joseph took me to Wal-Mart to get some groceries and then brought me back home. After doing more unpacking I went to sleep at 11 pm.

About an hour later, the landlord and her sons awake me about a missing TV. They ask if I heard anything and I tell them no. The landlord doesn't believe me and calls the police. She accuses me and the police ask me about the missing TV. I tell them everything and they recommend I find a place to stay. The only person I can get a hold of is Miss Sadie and she sends Dorrell to the house. As I was about to the leave, I ask the police about my $400 that I gave this woman for September rent. They said they can ask about it but they cannot force her to give it back to me. So, I did not get my money back and was forced to leave. Dorrell drove around for two hours looking for a place for me to stay. We drove from hotel to hotel with no luck until finally we found a Super Inn. I was exhausted. Dorrell helped me with my bags, I checked in, and finally slept.

The following morning, Dorrell picks me up for church and as we were on our way to church, his phone rings and it turns out that Darlene went to the church talking to the Pastor trying to scam the Pastor out of more money to pay for her 'stolen' TV. The Pastor says he wants to see us in the office immediately. We arrive at church, go to his office and I tell him the story.

I came to the conclusion that this Darlene was either nuts or a con artist. I believed she was both. After the meeting, I go into church and I was worshipping God like a mad woman because I was determined not to let the devil steal my praise. At the end of service, God worked it out that a lady from church allowed me to stay in her place without charging me for September due to my predicament. God is amazing.

The following day, I visited with the Pastor to tell him what happened and my intentions for being in Atlanta. He also prophesied that God was going to turn my shame around. He looked up Bipolar Disorder and asked me if I was showing symptoms of it. I confirmed the ones I did show. At the end of the meeting, he said he believed that I was not bipolar but having trouble releasing things. He said I allowed things to fester until I get an extreme reaction and also said I needed to learn how to respond by weighing the consequences of my actions because I was reacting to people and getting myself in trouble. Finally, he told me the definition of anger is unresolved issues. He said problems form when you don't close your issues. He reminded me that I needed to forgive my former church, which I did months ago. At the end of the discussion, he told me he didn't have a problem with me worshipping at his congregation, but only asked that I tell him directly if I encounter any problems.

I was so glad to be in Georgia and at the church. I really wanted to make a life down in Georgia but needed God's direction. After attending a service, the pastor laid out a plan of delegation and listed all the departments and who would report to who. This was a church of order; nothing like my previous church. I really wanted to stay in Georgia. I decided that I would ask the church to sponsor me.

I contacted the consulate first and it turns out that moving to Georgia is a bit more difficult than I thought. I started to question why God allowed me to come here. I believe that I was there to get my healing of my issues. I believed that I needed to be in a place that was slower and this was the case. I came to Georgia feeling like a failure because of all the things that went wrong in my life.

I then got an idea about how I can make money. I decide that I will create a retail store and e-store. I wanted to create a website where I would sell my skirts and the products of other vendors. I started to work on the idea and search for places to lease for my store. As I worked on the idea, I came to a few conclusions: my business is expensive to run, my prices are too high for my current clientele, I can't sew my own clothing because I do not own a machine, cutting table or serger, and I do not have a seamstress I am comfortable with. With this reality, I decided I would go back home to Canada humble and do more research.

While in Georgia I was blessed to meet a young man named Terry Gilmore at a McDonald's. I told him about Jesus and did a few bible studies with him. Finally, he decided to get baptized and got baptized before I left for Canada. It was so amazing.

Another person I was blessed to meet was a young man named Nathan, the founder of a company Apostolic Clothing. He happened to be doing the same thing that I was dreaming about. We had a long conversation and he had agreed to sell my clothing on his website and I would sell his clothing in Canada. On November 1, 2012, we had agreed to meet up before I left for Canada where he would give me some of his inventory. Then I got a message that he wanted to reschedule. Later I got an email saying he wanted to cancel the whole project because of advice he received from his pastor. When I read it, it sounded like he was being discouraged from doing business with me. I started to feel very depressed, sad, and beaten up. I took a walk and got to the highway overpass. It had a large fence on it and I remember standing there wishing the fence wasn't there so I could jump. It was only a dream.

I had another meeting with Pastor Woodstock Sr. and I felt so good. He encouraged me so much and told me that God was behind all my trials to make me turn back to God on a more intimate level. He also told me that I would not be returning to my old church and it was not my job to try and fix their church but just to move on. He told me that APC was my place of refuge and my new church. I was to make myself useful to them and serve. He then told me that my plan to help Gospel Rappers was a distraction and I was to leave that project alone. He also said that the devil had been distracting me from my real gifts. He said that I have been gifted to write, do poetry and maybe be a life coach but that devil was trying to steal my gifts and use it for his glory. Finally, he said, when I go home, I should try to establish a steady income and that God's delays are not his denials.

I was so thankful that I was able to come to Georgia because of the lessons I learned and the word I received that said I was not bipolar.

Chapter 5:
I Am Cleoni: I Am Bipolar

In the middle of November 2012, I came back to Toronto, Canada and started to feel like a failure again. I started to have suicidal thoughts but was encouraged by the word that Pastor Woodstock Sr. from Georgia gave me. The Lord blessed me with a free sewing machine. I only had to buy a new peddle which cost me $85. I was thankful. However, I was blessed to get a new job, a 9-5 and I was not happy. I questioned if it was the will of God. Then, I decided to go to APC and really worshipped God. I told a sister that I was having suicidal thoughts. She gathered some saints to pray for me and to bind the stronghold. One of the ministers said I was entertaining the thought. I was entertaining it because I felt like a failure. I wanted to do something that I was passionate about. I really needed help. I started to lose desire to try anymore. I wanted to give up on life. I was sick of poverty, living in a bedroom not an apartment, and failure. I felt sick and tired. I just wanted life to end. I begged Jesus to end my life because I was tired.

It was November 24, 2012 when I came to a revelation. I finally admitted that I had Bipolar Disorder. I remember looking in the mirror and saying, *"My name is Cleoni Crawford and I have Bipolar Disorder."* I felt liberated because I was accepting my disorder. I was no longer fighting it. I was accepting it. I was able to say it confidently, because I recognized that my bipolar disorder was not bigger than Jesus and this label would not stand in the way of my success. I was no longer going to be fearful of what people would say about me. I was more concerned what God had to say about me. As far as I was concerned, Jesus made me this way. This sickness will keep me humble. It will keep me on my knees so I don't lose my focus. I believed that God allowed Pastor Woodstock Sr. to make one error about me. He said I was not bipolar. If he had said I was, I would have tuned him out and claimed he was just like the rest and would have missed all the other prophecies he gave me. Furthermore, speaking to him made me realize that I had other issues that led up to the Bipolar Episodes. The way I handled stress needed to change. Also, I needed to stop allowing things to fester until I blew up. So, to solve these problems I decided to get some counselling and contacted Christine Blake.

Now that I had accepted that I was a Bipolar Christian, I felt free and started to share my testimony. I was cool with the label. I took the bus to meet my church bus in Scarborough since I still lived in Rexdale with my grandmother. While on the bus, I started to openly share my testimony about being bipolar. There was one woman who listened intently as she also had a mental illness. From this encounter, I chatted with her and then gave her Christine Blake's number for counselling. When I got to church, my new Pastor, Pastor Castro, preached a sermon that spoke to my heart called, *"God is trying to get your attention."* He said that God will use 5 ways to get your attention, 1. Voice, 2. Visions, 3. Vile Afflictions, 4. Vicarious Situations, and 5. Visitation from God. By the time he got to #3, I ran to the altar and sat down listening to the Pastor. I was convinced that God was speaking to me and telling me that I needed to become a licensed minister who runs a business. I was so thankful for this revelation. After service, I fellowshipped with people and would have conversations that did not feel forced. I was definitely more talkative than normal. Following this, I went downstairs to find the women fellowshipping in the kitchen preparing food. While there, my phone rings. I tell my mother the good news of my revelation and she accuses me of being sick. Then I speak to my brother and tell him he needs to get baptized. He ignores me and says he will do what the Bible tells him to do.

I started to post heavily on social media again. I would post various different photos of me travelling to different parts of the city. From someone looking in, the pictures did not connect. However, for me, the pictures were representations of where I went and how much favour I was about to receive. I would take photos of everything. I would take photos of my smoothies, my dinner, my workout, the dishes, and so much more. It was ridiculous when I look back. I was clearly manic but did not know it. This was the beginning to my Instagram posts. I would post photos of me meeting various strangers. I would post photos of musicians, the church, books I'm reading, screenshots and so much more. By this time, I had switched from the name the #VirtuousWoman to #JudahPraizes. Whenever I am manic, I would create a name based on how I was feeling. Also, during this time, I was watching many Tyler Perry movies featuring Madea. I started to feel like I was the real life Jamaican Madea. During this time, I would visit many malls and talk selfies of me in front of these stores. By taking a photo, it would show whether I approved of the store and if they were going to receive the blessing. There were times that if I disapproved of a store, I would spit on its window to signify that they were cursed. According to my revelations, the following organizations and stores were cursed: TD Bank, Bell, Bell Mobility, and McDonalds to name a few.

My beliefs had drastically changed. I would listen to a lot of music during this time as I travelled. To show the different types of songs I would listen to, I would take screenshots of them and post them on Instagram, Facebook and Twitter. I would post several times per day and it was getting crazy.

Finally, in February 2013, my mother decided to have me put into the hospital. She contacted the Justice of the Peace to have the police pick me up. I was furious because though sick, I didn't believe I belonged there. This time I stayed in the hospital for 6 days. I was not able to prove the doctors that I was well after the 3 days. It was horrible. They gave me drugs to calm me down and become more stable. While there I contacted the Psychiatric Patients Advocates Office to get out. They provided a representative that told me my rights. Finally I was released. I was once again upset at my mom. My grandmother had moved out of her condo and I did not have anywhere to stay.

For the first time in my life, I went to a shelter in Ajax. I was so thankful that I found a place to stay. However, the following day, the owners of the shelter decided to tell me that I had to leave. They did not give me an explanation. I was so angry I told them to call the police. When the police came, I threw the underwear that they gave me at them. I said I didn't need their charity and left the building. I crossed the street and did my lion dance asking for favour. I started to walk through Ajax calling friends and family looking for a place to stay to no avail. I was cold and Jack Frost was starting to affect my fingers. So, I found a building and went inside to get warm. I took the elevator to the top floor and sat in the stairwell. I was tired, so I fell asleep in the stairwell for a few minutes. Then, I contacted the Salvation Army and they gave me the number to the Muslim Welfare Home in Whitby. When I called them, they said they had room. Immediately, I got on a bus and went to Whitby.

I arrived in Whitby at the Muslim Welfare Home. This was weird for me being a Christian in a Muslim shelter. It turned out not to be too bad. I stayed in the shelter for 3 weeks. I would go to church from the shelter every Wednesday, Friday and Sunday. The people at the shelter would always compliment me about my clothing. Thankfully, nothing was ever stolen. However, while there, I was manic and would take many photos of the city at night and claim certain businesses were there to help me. I felt like Whitby was home. I felt like God was sending me there to settle down.

While there, I visited the MPP's office Christine Elliot looking for help and a job. I felt like I was being attacked and targeted by the police and needed help. So, I got the MPP to contact the police so I could tell them to leave me alone. They came and that is what I did. Then, I left. However, this did not stop the police from harassing me. They stopped me once I was jogging, in No Frills, and at the shelter. I was starting to feel like I was being targeted.

The second politician I visited was Jim Flaherty's office. I was so fed up with Canada at this point. I wanted to leave the country. I wanted to be a refugee. I wanted to start over. So, I walked to his office looking for help and when I arrived there, I had no energy. I begged them to help me become a refugee. Then, suddenly, I fainted and started to cry and shake. They called the ambulance and next thing I knew I was in the Lakeridge hospital in Oshawa.

The nurses at Lakeridge did not treat me well. I was still manic. They didn't tend to me and I felt like they were out to get me. So, I slipped out of the room and started to leave the hospital. I said this hospital was going to be judged by the Lord for how they were treating its Prophet. So, as I was leaving, I pulled the fire alarm and slipped out the door. The hospital went into lockdown and I ran fearfully praying I would not get caught. It was late at night when I left the hospital. I started to pray and walk down streets that I felt the Holy Ghost was leading me to. I did not know my way around Oshawa especially at that time at night. After hours of walking, I got to Mary Street and that is when I realized that God was with me. Mary was the name of my counsellor. As I walked down Mary Street, I felt a sense of peace.

I decided that I would look for a place in Oshawa. I went back to the shelter, continuing to look for a place to live. Finally, after 3 weeks, I left the shelter because I got a new place to stay in Pickering. I moved into a room for rent. It was really nice but I only lasted there for 2 weeks. I was manic and paranoid living there due to the Muslim temple across the street. I felt like the Muslim gods were attacking me. I remember not being able to sleep. I started packing my bags but soon realized this was the devil wanting me to be unstable and end up in another shelter. After talking to two friends, I started to unpack again. However, I started to cook in my landlord's kitchen and was told that it wasn't going to work out because I cooked too often. I was told to move. This was sad but I was also happy due to the spiritual attacks I was facing.

Slowly I was becoming more and more irritable. I didn't recognize it as being irritable but being misunderstood. I longed to be understood. I was losing friends and people were looking at me funny. I thought they were the problem. They just didn't have the same revelation as I did. They are the ones with the problem.

I remember being invited to a church sister's house to fellowship. I hadn't been invited out in a long time. I was really looking forward to hanging out. There was a discussion about relationships and everyone was giving their opinions. I decided to share my opinion. I remember one of the brother's respond to my comment by indirectly dissing me. I was so hurt by it that I got up and walked out. My friend and the host ran after me but I was too hurt. I was tired of being misunderstood and disrespected. I shouted at them and told them to leave me alone. I also used some profanity. I was tired of being misunderstood.

Canadians were hurting me and no one understood me. This was the last time that I was going to be disgraced. I was done with Canada and longed for my second family, my DUPC family and Terry in Atlanta, Georgia. Angry and frustrated, I decided to walk through Oshawa to the train station. I didn't know where I was going. I depended on the Holy Spirit to guide me. While walking, I remember the city being filled with fruit flies. I deemed this as confirmation that Oshawa and all its residents were living on a cursed land. To me, this explained why I was dissed. I was a prophet who was being rejected by Oshawa. To me, the demons of Oshawa recognized that I was in their city and used that church brother to offend me. In my mind, it made sense. Therefore, I, the Prophet, or so I thought, would curse the land by walking through it for the last time. Finally, I arrived at the Oshawa GO centre and saw the VIA Rail sign. I took this as a sign that I would be taking the VIA rail and AMTRAK to Atlanta, Georgia. I was going to ride the bus but did not have any money on my PRESTO card. So, I decided to take the GO train without paying. I knew this was wrong but I needed to get back to church and out of this cursed city as soon as possible.

In May 2013, I acted on my thoughts to leave Canada for Atlanta, Georgia. However, it did not go how I planned. I went there with limited resources and was trying to move there. I stayed in a motel for about a week with no trouble. While there I was manic and did not know it. I posted numerous photos and videos on Instagram. When I say I posted many photos; I posted pictures of everything I saw. Everything had a meaning. I continued the same antics that I did in Toronto. I was delusional. I would talk to everyone I met. I would call them Prophets or Prophetesses depending on my inner checklist. I would identify people by colours or numbers. I was strongly into biblical numerology. If they were wearing red, they were a prophet, blue, an apostle, white, pure, or black for the black Jews. Also, numbers like 1, 2, 4, 8, and 12 were all good numbers. One was for unity, 2 for marriage, 4 for balance, 8 for new beginnings, 12 for divine government. These numbers guided me and how I related to people. My senses were hyper sensitive. Everything I encountered had a meaning, even magazines were prophesying to me and about me. I went to the church and they provided love for me.

However, while at the motel, I ran out of money and called the church for help. I asked if they could put me up and they declined. I was really hurt. However, when I told them I had no food, they provided me with a basket full of food. The pastor told me that I needed to go back to Canada. I did not want to go. Canada had been stressing me out. During this time, I stayed on the sofa at Terry Gilmore's, my new friend.

The family showed me kindness and I was truly appreciative of their support. I decided that I would host a concert to raise money. I met an artist who I thought would perform. Terry and I started to try to sell tickets that I had printed at Kinko's and were unsuccessful. Things weren't working out for, so I finally decided to take the advice of the pastor and go home. I came back to Canada.

Upon my return, I moved back home to my mother's place. I was saddened but still manic. I decided that I would do a concert here in Canada featuring this artist in Buffalo named Kyria. To do this, I decided to travel to Buffalo to meet Kyria and talk business. I went downtown to Kinko's and bought supplies for the business cards I would be making and other things. I had about four Kinko bags. From there, I went to the bus station on Bay St. and boarded the greyhound to Buffalo. When I got to the border, the border officers told us to leave the bus for inspection. I told the officer that I was going to Buffalo for a business trip. They looked at my bags and thought I was trying to flee the country. I was not allowed to board the bus to continue my trip to Buffalo. They put me in the holding cell as they checked me out and took my fingerprints. This was embarrassing.

Eventually, they informed me that they kept me so long because someone with my last name was wanted and they wanted to make sure it wasn't me. I was so upset and offended. Next they said that I should go back home. I decided I would stay in Niagara Falls because I was in a good mood. I travelled to downtown Niagara Falls by foot with my bags and suitcase. Unfortunately, it started to rain and all my bags got soaked.

I made it to a Karaoke bar called the Beer Garden. It was outdoors. My mood was very high. I had so much energy that I just wanted to sing. So, I went on the stage and I sang in the rain. I sang Whitney Houston's song, **"I wanna dance with somebody."** I felt electric. I left the stage and went into the audience and started to dance to the people singing. Then, this drunken man, Norman, came towards me and tried to dance with me. He offered to pay for my drink; I took orange juice. Soon after it was the last round and then then Beer Garden was closed. Norman asked me if I had a place to stay and I didn't. So, he offered to have me stay at his place. I went to his home and it was a mess. However, I was homeless, so I pushed passed the mess. I stayed in his bed and went to sleep.

The next morning, I said I would go back to the border and try to cross because I had a return ticket to Toronto from Buffalo. He followed me to the border and I met with an officer who also denied me entrance. I was livid and I snapped. I started to rip pages out of a book and spit and swear and carry on. It was bad. Then seven US border officers arrived and put a mask over my head. They tackled me down to the ground and handcuffed me. They took off my shoes, and cavity searched me. It was degrading. Then they drove me to the Canadian border barefoot in the rain. It was horrible. I walked to the border singing loudly the Canadian National Anthem. I was told to quiet down by a female officer. So I threw a book at her and claimed that she was speaking to the next Governor General. I continued to sing and another officer told me to quiet down. I looked at her and spat at the desk in front of her. She threatened me and told me that if I spat again, I would be arrested. I spat again and I was arrested. She claimed that I had spit on her. I did not. They put me in a holding cell. I started to sing to calm myself down. I started to rap curse words about the officers. Then suddenly, I fainted and started to have a seizure. They called the ambulance and they came and checked me out. I was barely conscious. They didn't care. They took me to jail. I was in the Niagara Falls Regional Police Station for the night.

The following day, I went before the judge and was sentenced to prison for my assault. They sent me to the women's prison, Vanier Centre for Women. They stripped me naked and had me shower in front of the guards. Then, they returned the shackles back on my feet and arms and we went to my jail cell. I was still manic. I started to bang on the jail cell screaming, *"Let me out, I'm innocent."* I kept doing this for a long time until the guards returned and took me to a private cell in the mental health ward. They thought I was crazy. My cell had a steel door with a metal slot for food. I continued to yell and then finally went to sleep but was happy to find a Bible in the cell.

The next morning, I started to rap and sing again. They called me the songbird. They would feed me through the slot. They would always keep peeping on me to see what I was doing. I became annoyed at this so decided to use the bible to make papier-mache. I ripped out pages of the bible and used water to paste them onto my jail cell. Then, I took toilet paper and covered the window of my jail cell. One of the guards came by to ask what I was doing, I replied, *"F**k off, I'm working."* I continued to plaster the bible around my cell. This made me happy. The following day, a guard who I called a racist came by and wanted to know what I was up to. I did not like this guard. I decided that the next time he came to deliver something for me; I would have a surprise for him. So I put my poop in the little slot. The next time he came to my cell, he found my poop and started to scream and swear. I laughed. They came into my room and got me to clean off my masterpiece from the walls. I was pissed. I started to rap insults at the guards and then, I fainted and started to have a seizure. They noticed it and called the doctor. They dragged me out of my cell and started to check my pulse. I could hear them but I could not respond. I would keep shaking so they called the ambulance. I was transferred to the Oakville Trafalgar Memorial Hospital.

When I woke up I was in the hospital bed with a guard watching me. They had shackled my feet to the bed so I could not escape. To go to the washroom, they would shackle my feet together and let me waddle to the restroom. It was horrible and degrading. While in the hospital I would speak to the guards and tell them about my business ideas. They would commend me on them. I was very talkative and very manic. However, I was getting better. I stayed in the hospital chained up for 5 days and then finally went back to prison. I remained there for 2 days and then went before the judge. I did not have a lawyer and the CMHA (Canadian Mental Health Association of Niagara Falls) came to see me in St. Catherine's. They spoke on my behalf and I was released from jail and put on probation for 1 year. I had a criminal record. Both my mother and Norman were there. My mother wanted me to come back home. I came back home with her temporarily for a few days. However, I was starting to miss Niagara Falls, so I went back to Norman's place in Niagara Falls. He said I could live there and stay on his couch and I was fine with that.

    Being released and living in Niagara Falls was great. I was so grateful to be released. It was really hard being locked up. Now that I was released, I had to return back to the prison to pick up my stuff. While on the Go Bus, the #12, from Niagara Falls to Vanier Centre for Women in Milton, I noted the bus number 2374 and started to decode it. The digits added up to 16 and 168 when multiplied and somehow, I came to the number 15. This was a confirmation to me that I was in the perfect will of God. You see this is what I had been doing. I had been decoding numbers wherever I went and these numbers either were blessings or curses. If the numbers added up to numbers like 3, 5, 9, or 13, I knew I was safe and hence could board that bus or deal with the person. I arrived and picked up my belongings from prison and was so thankful to be out of that place. I was really hungry so I went to the McDonald's across the street. While there, eating my burger, I met this couple. I started to tell them they were blessed and that I was going to bless them with a free hotel stay at the hotel that I was going to host my event at. They were happy to hear this. The thing was that I did not have any money to pay for this hotel. How was I going to pay for such a gift? You see, when manic, I just assume that anything is possible because, I'm a millionaire in process.

After I finished eating, I left and went back to Niagara Falls. I truly loved it there. Specifically, I loved going to the Beer Garden for their Karaoke. It kept me fuelled. Also, the attendees loved my singing. Niagara Falls was really good to me. The people were friendly and this made me hate Toronto much more. Another good thing that was happening at the time was that I found out that The 700 Club TV show was interested in my testimony. I just knew this was what I needed. So, I started to get myself comfortable in Niagara Falls by making note of all the businesses that were in the city. By the evening, I decided to go to the Beer Garden for Karaoke. I called it my coming out party. I sung, **"I wanna dance with somebody"** by Whitney Houston and **"Black or White"** by Michael Jackson. There was an 8-year-old kid with spiked hair that was grooving to the songs. He along with the crowd loved my singing. This was confirmation to me that this was truly home.

While in Niagara Falls, I started to plan a conference that would be about raising awareness for mental health. It was going to be a conference featuring American and Canadian organizations hosted in Niagara Falls at the Legion. I created a list of at least 35 people and organizations that would take part in this conference. I would talk about raising awareness for bipolar and how people and organizations can provide support to them. It would also offer awards to recognize organizations that are providing great support to people with bipolar.

Though living in Niagara Falls, I decided that I would still go to my church in Pickering. I considered Toronto as cursed, but not Pickering or Mississauga was cursed; they were safe zones. It was Sunday June 16, 2013 when I decided to go to church for Sunday service. It was Father's Day. I took my roommate Norman with me. It was a 3-hour trip on the Go Transit. It was expensive so I got my roommate to pay for it. He had been helping me out until I got on my feet. We arrived at church and it was Father's Day. The sermon was called *"Real Fathers Always There."* It was a powerful sermon. Norman really enjoyed the service. I brought him along to show my church that I was not crazy. I wanted him to explain that he was working as my assistant and believed that I was fine. Though I told myself I was fine, I knew I was still manic. After service, we took the train back to Niagara Falls. I was happy to be home. Sadly, all good things come to an end. Though I wanted to continue to stay with Norman, his brother found out I was staying there and said I needed to move out. I contacted my mother and moved back to Toronto.

Chapter 6:
My Saving Grace

It was uncomfortable living at home with my mother. I found her to be controlling and she didn't believe that I was okay. She thought that I was manic. Despite, this, I decided to focus on my new businesses that I wanted to create. I created a list of 27 items on my to-do list. One of those items was to sue Ascend, the previous store that I was in but was kicked out due my mental illness. I was still angry about it and wanted justice. Though I wanted to sue Ascend, they were not the only people on my hit list. There were numerous people. I find when I think back, when manic, I always want to sue someone for justice. The main people on that list were the Toronto Police, my previous employers at the Ontario Public Service, and various doctors and nurses that have treated me poorly. While manic, I continued to travel around the city and take various photos of places I visited. Due to my posting, my mother became aware of how many posts I would post. Sometimes in one day, I could post 100 times. I didn't think there was anything wrong with that since everything in my mind had a meaning. She would complain about my activity and I finally got fed up and decided to do something about it.

On Friday July 5, 2013, to prove that I was fine, I decided to go to CAMH to get my hospital records that would prove that I did not need medication. However, when I went there, they decided to do an assessment on me. I explained to a doctor that I was an entrepreneur that has bipolar and only wanted to get my hospital records. I also showed him how focused I was and that I only wanted to plan my businesses and be left alone. Sadly, none of this mattered. I was a nigger that couldn't have a business. I must be ill. I was told that they would be keeping me.

I was livid. I started to complain and scream that I was not ill. They called the security guards on me and had me strapped to a hospital bed. They gave me a needle and I cried. Eventually, I calmed down and fell asleep. When I awoke it was 12:30am and I was still in the emergency department.

The following day, they sent me upstairs to the PICU (Psychiatric Intensive Care Unit) to stay. I did not realize how long I would stay up there. While there, I requested that I get my phone, which had my music. My music was my therapy, my music therapy. I could not sleep so I asked for my music. My nurse, Monique, denied me my music; I was pissed. However, she offered me plenty of Ativan, which I explained was not good for me as it caused me to have seizures. She didn't care. She explained that my phone had a camera on it and cameras were not permitted on the unit. I explained to her that my camera was not working. That didn't matter. Instead, I watched her hand a patient a substitute cigarette for his nerves or his therapy. This was so frustrating. Why did smokers have more rights than I did?

While there, I would journal a lot. There was nothing that I could do so I would journal and plan my business for when I got out of the hospital. I wrote in my journal that since CAMH was unwilling to help me, I would help myself. I would stay at CAMH till I got four things: 1) ODSP, 2) Subsidized housing at 10 San Romanoway, 3) My lawsuit and 4) An open apology from Queen's Park. I refused to take medication because as far as I was concerned, I did not belong there. So once again, they called the security officers and they strapped me down again. I lay on the bed helpless and angry.

How could they do this to me? I was intelligent. I was not crazy. I did not deserve to be treated like this. This unit had no windows and no sunlight.

While in this unit, I couldn't sleep. I was offered Ativan and I refused it and asked for my music. The nurses kept telling me to get some rest. I assured them if I wasn't getting my music as requested, I wouldn't be sleeping. I had not slept for two full days when finally, I was given access to music. I was given the opportunity to use the computer on the other side for a few minutes. I used the computer to listen to music because I realized how much it meant to me. I was grateful. I finally got to sleep.

The day before I was going to be re-assessed I was excited; however, it was short lived. I got into an argument with one of the nurses, Nurse Dan to be exact. He pissed me off, so I spit on him. The security was called for this and I was given a needle and put into isolation. The nurse that was assigned to me the next morning said that I was still going to be re-assessed, and that if I played nice, I might go home. She happened to be a Christian. I decided in preparation for the meeting, that I would read every scripture about LOVE and MERCY until they arrive. I was so confident that I would be going home.

I met with the doctors, Dr. Glenda Horowitz and resident Dr. Chen, and they claimed I was too ill. So they didn't release me and extended my stay at CAMH by giving me a form 3. I cried and did not understand why. I decided it was time to contact my PPAO (Psychiatric Patients Advocate's Office) representative and find out my rights. The representative came and told me that I had the right to a hearing. I got a lawyer and decided I wanted a hearing. While in PICU, I became so stressed that I started to have seizures. I had 24 seizures in the 16 days that I was at CAMH. My experience at

CAMH on this occasion was horrible. They took away my music again and did not give me access to sunlight.

While there I started to develop theories about my predicament. I started to believe that the principalities Jezebel and Pharmakos were out to get me. I believed that my illness was both spiritual and chemical. While in the ward, I would sing and praise God. Some people liked it and others didn't. One night, one of the patients asked me to sing to him so he could fall asleep. I discerned that there were demons that were affecting him. So, I prayed and started to sing. He fell asleep and later thanked me and told me that he had not been able to sleep like that in a long time

Then, one day, a very large fat Indian man came into the unit. Apparently, he was a UofT graduate getting his PhD. We started to talk and then I realized that your intelligence did not have to do with your mental illness. One night after midnight, he came to me and started to speak in this deep dark voice. He said the following, *"I know who you are."* I responded, *"Who am I?"* He continued, *"You are one those Christians."* Right away, I responded, *"What is your name?"* He continued, *"I am Zeus."* I responded, *"In the name of Jesus, come out of him!"* He screamed, rolled his back and faced me again. He laughed. I said, *"What is your name?"* He said, *"I am Zorastus."* I replied, *"In the name of Jesus, come out of him!"* He screamed and fell to the floor curled in a ball and started to sob. That day, I came to the realization that not all of these people in mental hospital were chemically ill but some were spiritual possessed.

Finally, it came the time for my hearing. I was all prepared and despite this, our request was denied. I was so depressed. However, the doctors made the decision to have me get some sunlight and go to the General unit on the other side. I was so thankful. There is nothing to do in PICU except colouring and I was sick of that. The general unit had a piano, TV, books, daily workshops and day passes. I would play the piano and sing **"Lean on me"** at the top of my lungs. It was so good to have music back. People loved my singing and some of the patients would sing along. I only stayed another week and was finally released on July 24, 2013.

After being released from the hospital, I reluctantly moved back to my mother's home. Though I knew she loved me, I grew distrustful of her because she was responsible for me being hospitalized on numerous occasions. Despite this, I was thankful that she provided me a place to live. I slept in her bed but had my stuff in suitcases because I did not have space for my belongings. I felt like I was still homeless. I longed for a place of my own. I longed for independence.

Though I came out of the hospital full of energy and promise about my business endeavors, my mood slowly decreased. It was gradual. First, it started with feelings of being a failure in my 30s. Then, I started to grieve all the losses I had. As the days passed, I started to be sad and then clinically depressed. I had no job, no volunteer opportunities and no real business opportunities. I no longer thought that I could actually do all the things I thought I could do. I was hopeless. My life looked bleak. My mood became very dark. All I did was watch television, eat and sleep. Sometimes, I would not shower. I found no reason to put on house clothing. I would stay in my pajamas for days. Along with my inability to put on clothes, I started to refuse food. I lost my enthusiasm for life. Like, what was the point? I'm going to be a failure anyhow.

If it had not been for church, I would have no reason to leave my home. I did not have many friends and was not getting any calls to hang out. The only thing I had was church. Though I had my church, I still became depressed and hopeless. When I would leave my home, I would start to think about dying. I wanted to die. Yes, I said it, I wanted to die. If I was going to be a failure, I no longer wanted to live. It was a struggle each week to make it to church but still I went. Though, I went to church, I would come home with lingering thoughts of death.

I started to look up ways on the Internet how to die. There was drowning myself, jumping off the bridge, hanging myself, overdosing on pills, or getting a gun. I remember starting to reason with each choice. How I could kill myself quickly.

The first method I seriously considered was hanging myself. When my mother would leave and go to work, I found packing wire/rope and tied it to the bannister to support myself and then I started to cry as I put the rope around my neck. I kept stepping down the stairs, step by step, in an effort to kill myself. The pressure of the rope started to tighten and cut through my neck. I was starting to dangle. The rope was getting tighter and tighter around my neck. The blood started to rush to my brain. The pressure became unbearable. I jumped back up the stairs. I can't do this, I reasoned. Though I tried it, it was not the last time. I would continue to try and stop because it was too painful. I knew I wanted to die but I did not want to die a painful death.

Another method I tried was something that I learned about while watching Criminal Minds. One episode was about teens hanging themselves with a scarf over a doorknob. I knew this would be painful. Despite this, I tried it several times. I made a noose by looking it up on the Internet and put the scarf around my neck. Then, I tied the opposite end around the doorknob and started to go limp. I really wanted this to work. However, once I started to feel the blood rush up my brain, I gave up. I needed to find a new way to kill myself.

As I would go to church and cross the highway 401, the highway of heroes, along Whites Road, I would look over the bridge at all the fast moving cars. I would think to myself, what if I just jumped? What if I could just do it? It would be fast and all I need is the courage to jump. I think I could do this, I thought. However, a thought would come to stop me. I would think to myself, *"Cleoni, if you could only just get to the church, everything would be alright."* So time and time again, this would be the saving grace. I would go to church and though depressed, I would have the strength to live for one more day. I couldn't picture my life more than a day. The future was too much. One day while crossing the bridge along Whites Road, I started to look over the bridge. I was really starting to contemplate jumping. I took off my shoes and started to bend over and then I put my shoes back on and continued to go to church. I thought, what would my church think of me? Then, a police car pulls up to me as I walked to church. The officer calls me and asks me if I was okay. I told him I was and was just on my way to church. He said that they received a call that a woman was thinking of jumping. I lied and said I was just looking at the cars because I had a hard day but I'm good now. I knew if I didn't answer correctly, I would be back in the mental hospital, so I was careful with my words. They let me go and I vowed to never try to jump off that bridge again.

However, that was not the last time I tried to kill myself. The next method I considered was getting a gun. This would be the quickest method possible. I only would need to have the courage to pull the trigger. I searched on the Internet for a gun. I found several gun shops but they all required that you had a license. I knew I did not want to go through getting a license. I then thought about going to a gun range. I called one that was out of town and asked about their procedure. I started to think that I would go there, rent the gun and then kill myself. I asked the price and sadly it was out of my budget. So, I had to think of another method. The next method was to drown myself. I searched on the Internet to find certain lakes that I could go to drown myself. I found a lake downtown and told myself that I was going to go in the night while everyone was sleeping. I lay out my clothing on the bed. I told myself that this was it. I'm going to kill myself. Then, later that day, I receive a call. I started to tell them how sad I was and that I wanted to kill myself. They encouraged me to keep fighting. They spoke to my spirit and my spirit heard it. I told myself that I was not going to kill myself that day. However, the feelings kept lingering. As I would travel, I remember being at the Sheppard Station and telling myself that I would jump in front of the train. Each time I would take a step closer to the yellow caution line. I would hear the training coming. My heart would start to race. *"Just jump"*, I told myself. *"It's coming. Don't give the train operator a chance to see you jump. Just jump,"* I told myself. I breathed in deeply and braced myself. Then I sunk down and stepped back. I couldn't do it. Though I did not do it that day, I would still go through this process whenever I was in the subway.

Days, weeks, and months would pass and the thoughts would increase. I finally decided that it was time I got some help. I started to look up support groups for people with mental illnesses. I found Mood Disorders Association of Ontario at Eglington and Yonge and decided I would go. I went to the meeting and was given the chance to talk about my feelings. I remember listening to the various individuals and being able to identify with the stories. It was finally my chance to talk about I remember crying as I spoke. I told them about my suicidal ideations and they offered to speak to me after the meeting. I stayed back and told them about my attempts. They gave me a few numbers and told me about a one on one service that they offered. I decided to take them up on the offer. I would continue to go to the weekly meetings. Week by week I would feel a little bit better but I was still suicidal. I attended a few one-on-one sessions with a social worker. She asked if I was on medication. I told her that I wasn't. I was referred to a psychiatrist and decided to go. He was friendly and from the West Indies. He talked a lot but I liked him. He told me about Lithium and the side effects. I told him that I wanted to think about it. I went home and went to Google and looked it up and read about the side effects. Though there were side effects, I finally decided to take the medication. So it was settled, I was now on Lithium.

The more I attended the meetings, the better I felt. I started to make friends with a few people from the group. I was becoming a regular. I also started to go the Christian Counseling Services on Carlton Avenue and met a Christian Counselor named Mary. She was so friendly. I started to attend weekly. Coupled with the weekly sessions at Mood Disorders, with my counselor and my new medication, I started to feel better.

Then one day in October 2013, it dawned on me. I think I found my purpose. I now know why I was given Bipolar. I was supposed to help others. I decided that I wanted to be a Christian Counselor. I decided that I was going to ask Canada Christian College about their program. I asked about their program and found it interesting. Then, I told Mary my counselor about this and she told me she could refer me to her professor to do an informational interview. I called his office and got an interview. At the interview, I asked him many questions about the profession and the process that he recommended. He did not recommend Canada Christian Colleges because he said it was not accredited. So I decided that I would consider going back. I researched and discovered that I needed to upgrade my degree to an Honours bachelor and take some psychology courses in order to get a Masters. I thought about this and decided that I would put this on hold. I could not afford to go back to school and did not automatically qualify. So I decided to look into the Second Careers and unfortunately, this program only covered 2-year programs maximum and did not include postgraduate programs. I was saddened and was back to square one.

While attending the weekly sessions at MDAO, the facilitator discussed a free program at George Brown for people with mental illness and/or Addiction issues. She said it was a transition program to help people transition to go back to school or work. I decided that I would go for the information session. While there I saw one of the members from my weekly support group. It made me smile. I learned about the program and decided that I would apply. One thing that stood out for me was one of the testimonials from a Muslim woman named Amal. She expressed how thankful she was for TPE and how much it changed her life. I spoke to her after the session and she encouraged me to apply. With that exchange, I decided that I would apply. I applied and was admitted into the program and was ecstatic. The program was going to start in January of 2014 and was at the St. James Campus. Though I got in, I was worried that I was not going to be admitted in because of my suspension in 2008 and not having a psychiatric assessment. I decided that I would tread cautiously and play nice.

Chapter 7:
Happy or So I Thought

It was January 2014 and I started the Transition to Post-Secondary Education program (TPE for short) and was so excited. For the first time in a long time, I was given the chance to interact with high functioning individuals with mental illness who were trying to move forward with their life. This was so encouraging. I had great teachers. There were three teachers that stood out: Jaswant, Tenniel and Kate. Jaswant taught a course called Demystifying Mental Health and this really spoke to me. Kate taught a course about the Personal Narrative and writing our life. This course gave us the ability to write about our life and speak our truth. I fell in love with this course. Then, there was Tenniel. She was a black woman that taught about Psychology in Adult Development. She did not only teach me but she inspired me. She got me to think bigger and encouraged me. It was great to see a black woman that I could identify with.

The more I attended the classes, the more I would improve. My life was changing. The depression had faded and I had a reason to leave my home daily. My medication was working, my life had meaning and I was starting to make new friends.

In February of 2014, I found a new place; or more to the point, it found me. I qualified for ODSP and had more disposable income. I was looking for a place in Scarborough to be close to my church when I found this cute little place close to Malvern for only $500. It was tiny but it was good. I decided I would think about it. After finding a bigger place that was $600 but was shared I decided that I would take the first place. Unfortunately, when I called them back within one hour, the place was taken. I was so sad because I had even got a money order for $500 to pay my deposit but it was too late.

My mother and I decided that we would check one more place out at 7:30 pm but we had some time to spare so we decided to go to her friend's house to spare some time. While there, we met her brother and sister in law that was visiting. We chatted and I mentioned that I was looking for a place and was going to check one out later that evening. The gentleman mentioned that he had a place available for rent. He said we could go and check it out.

When I arrived at the house, I was blown away. It was a basement apartment with one of the largest kitchens I had seen in a long time. It was so clean and the cupboards were white and spotless. It was carpeted and had a cute living room, spacious bathroom and bedroom. I told him enthusiastically, that I would take the place. We returned back to my friend's house and I told them how excited I was about the place. They told me the rent was $750. I was disappointed because my budget was $600. Though it was lower than their price, they accepted it. I was so thankful because I now had my own apartment. Life was looking good for me.

It had been a while since I had been active in church. I was faithful in my church attendance as I never missed a service but I was not involved in ministry. I was a part of media ministry for a brief stint but due to my mental illness, I insulted a few of the members. I was at a new church and I had been a member for about a year and a half and already people saw my mentally ill side. Still, I was trying to rebuild myself. People noticed the changes and could see improvement. They would tell me that and I knew it was the case. Life was good despite my mental illness.

Black History Month was approaching and the church was doing a play and I was interested in taking part. A church brother and sister were in charge of putting this play together. It was a monologue and the brother thought I would be good for the female part. I loved drama and I was selected for the part. There were whispers about me being selected because I guess they thought I was too crazy. Who knows? Despite this, I was so excited to get back in ministry. I practiced my lines for hours and when it was time for the show, I performed and was told I did a phenomenal job. It was about a broken woman who had been raped and she was telling her story of pain. I nailed it. People truly felt the emotion I conveyed and were proud of me. I was proud of myself. Who knows what the future could hold? Only time would tell.

I was really enjoying my life at the present and was thankful. I was readmitted back in the media team doing the audio-visuals for the projector. I was seen as one of the best in the media room and when a special service was happening, they would count on me for it. It felt good to be useful again. Not only were things going good at church, life was great at school. I made many friends and was doing well in school. Also, I just found out about a program called Laughing Like Crazy hosted by MDAO. This was a 16-week program that taught you how to turn your mental health experiences into jokes. I had some experiences that I could share. I started to attend the sessions on a weekly basis and slowly started to grow comfortable with my painful experiences. I was able to laugh at myself. It's not always the easiest thing to do when you've been through a lot of garbage. As the weeks progressed, I had learned how to be quite the funny character.

It was March 2014 and the Academy Awards aka the Oscars was on the television and this is when I heard the song that changed my life. The beat was pumping and then comes Pharrell Williams and his hit song **"Happy"** being played. The performance was phenomenal. I got up from the sofa and started to dance. I hadn't felt like this in a while. The song was infectious. I danced and danced and truly felt happy. Once the performance was done, I searched for the music video and played it over and over again. I also downloaded it on iTunes and played this song over and over again while I sung the lyrics. The song spoke to me and become the anthem of my life.

Months later, I came up with an idea. I knew what my passion would be. I wanted to create a talk show that raised awareness for mental health. I wanted to showcase the stories of survivors. I wanted to show people that mental illness does not have to make us sad but we could be happy. That is how I came up with the name of my show, HappyHome42. The 42 came from an inspirational movie I had watched called 42 about the baseball player Jackie Robinson. I chose the word "*Home*" to signify that mental illness should be able to be talked about at home because it was a safe space. There were two individuals that meant a lot to me, Jackie Robinson and Pharrell Williams. I wanted to create a show that would be life changing. These two individuals were legends in my book and I wanted my show to be legendary and ground-breaking just like these two individuals.

After coming up with the idea to create a talk show, I decided to create a website called #IAMCLEONI. It was created in a few days and it had information about my past interviews and my new project. It also had links to all my social media accounts and a fundraiser link.

However, within days, it started again. I started to post on social media a lot. Whenever I am becoming manic, I start to post a lot on social media about everything. For example, on May 3, 2014, within

2 hours, I had taken 199 photos and posted 67 in one day. However, my posts usually had one theme. This time the theme was the **Happy** song from Pharrell. I wanted to show the world that I was truly happy. Little did I know that I was becoming manic. People started to notice. I had a long-time friend call me who had rejected me when I became ill last year. However, we had become friends again. To me, I felt like she doubted me and didn't understand me. She asked me if I was taking my medication. Despite what she thought, I was taking it but it just wasn't working.

I was becoming psychotic. I started to write in my journal that I thought that God had called me to be 1 of 4 of the greatest Apostles and Prophets in the globe. As far as I was concerned, God was about to make me a billionaire. However, in order to become a billionaire, I needed to build my team. I started to befriend a few brothers at church and told them that we would work together on different projects depending on their skillsets. I remember telling one brother that I considered my new best friend that we were going to start a rap group. With the other brother, I said we should start a basketball tournament.

Though the basketball tournament was a good idea, it was not well thought out. As per me becoming a rapper, this was just insane. However, in my eyes, it just made sense. I could rhyme a bit so I must be a rapper. In my mind, it was just that easy. The next thing I started to do was call various people I met directly or indirectly online or through their music.

For instance, I felt that Pharrell Williams was a prophet and I wanted the world to know that I knew. I would make various posts with Pharrell's album cover for the song **Happy**. It was used as banners and in collages; it was used everywhere. There must have been at least 100 posts about Pharrell and him being a prophet or connecting it to my new talk show. I would tag Pharrell in various posts in hopes that he would respond to me.

I posted about everything. I posted about books I was reading, food I ate, the various places I travelled, Google searches and its screenshots, people who were following me, people's Instagram profile pages. I was the queen of the screenshot. I even posted the private conversations that took place between my media team. I did not know that I was becoming ill but when I think back, I was truly ill. Due to my behavior, I was removed from the media team. However, on social media, I was getting numerous followers from everywhere. This was validation for me. The new followers told me that I was okay and that I was doing all that was necessary to get my talk show up. On the other hand, due to church members that were concerned about my obsessive behavior on social media, I thought I was being attacked and misunderstood. To comfort myself, I would play the **Happy** song over and over again. I needed to tell myself that I was happy. Eventually, all the accusations started to affect me. I started to post about Pharmakos and Jezebel being responsible for the death of my aunt and sister. I was determined to see them and the illuminati destroyed. So, I would post about the illuminati through videos and posts of code that I deemed to be speaking to me. I would become very harsh with the illuminati and their supposed followers. It was really bad. I was truly obsessed.

Then the next meltdown happened. I was tired and wasn't sleeping. I started to make videos of me crying and lying on the ground in an attempt to get help; however, it never came. So I contacted 911 and told them about my issue and they hung up on me stating that my issue wasn't serious enough. So, I copied the post showing that I called them and they denied me the ambulance to come to my house. I also posted a photo of me lying on the ground as if I was about to die. I was desperate but still no one responded to my posts. No one came to my aid. In my mind everyone was persecuting me. I did not know what else to do.

Another thing I did during this time was travel around the city. I would walk everywhere because I believed that I was like Abraham in the bible. In the bible it says that Abraham was given dominion and an inheritance wherever his foot touched. So I would walk through malls, hotels, supermarkets, pharmacies, grocery stores and even the Toronto Stock Exchange because I believed that God would give me ownership and/or favour in these places. In my eyes, I was a prophetess and my job was to bless and curse. However, not everyone believed this. There were people in my church that believed I was delusional. One brother actually used the pulpit to speak against me. I was so offended. I immediately 'unfriended' him.

Despite my mental state, I was still able to get some things done. I was focused on getting my talk show developed so I went to the Daystar Group and met with the manager Carlton about my show. He introduced me to the producer Melica. She was going to help me make my show a reality. She also had a mental illness and was inspired by the idea and was excited to help with this project. I would meet with her weekly and together we would work on the details.

As I would travel on the bus, I would strive to build a team of people that I could add to my team. I would talk to complete strangers who I felt led to speak to and tell them about myself and let them know that I thought they were prophets or apostles because I wanted to build a team of prophets and apostles for my future business. As relationships evolved, I would revise my list of people I thought I would work with me as future guests on the show or as part of the team. For example, I met two young boys that I thought were prophets due to the colour of clothing that they were wearing. They were both wearing black and red. To me, this combination meant they were prophets. I met each boy on two separate occasions. One boy I met in the Jane-Finch area playing basketball with friends. I told him that he was a prophet and could be on television. He thought it was interesting. I took his number and address and contacted his mother and spoke to her about it and she agreed to allow her son to be on the show. The second boy I met on the Finch bus while travelling home. He was wearing black and red and had a black hat. Black meant he was a black Jew and red meant he was a prophet. This young man was Filipino. We chatted and then exchanged numbers. His family came by my home and we discussed the TV show and they liked the idea. They decided that they would allow their son the chance to be a part of the television show.

Though I was being productive, I was also posting things online that were questionable. I was posting various screenshots of people I met on Instagram and offering them jobs in exchange for clothing at first and later as we grew $100K per year. I took the bus and train from Toronto via Durham to Niagara Falls. While in Toronto, I visited various places like hotels, restaurants, malls, and much more. While in the lobby of a hotel, I would make a reservation by faith that I would stay there in the future. I went to the Hilton, the Sheraton, and also the Fairmont Royal York.

One night while in the lobby of the Fairmont Royal York, I was using their Wi-Fi and sitting on the sofa, when I was approached by a security guard named Tyler and asked to leave. Suddenly, in a panic, I fainted and had a seizure. They called the ambulance and I told them all I wanted was a room. I was denied a room and told that I should leave. After the ambulance left, I shouted that I would be suing them and left the hotel. I didn't understand why I was being treated so unfairly. However, I was manic and did not see it. I left the hotel and continued to post about my experience, the illuminati, mammon, and much more.

Everywhere I went; I would see police and assume that they were looking for me. I was convinced because one night I posted at Bay station on the subway platform and then all of a sudden I saw police come downstairs to where I was. So I quickly, went upstairs and left the station. I posted another post about it when I got to the Tim Horton's outside the station. Once done, I turned my phone on airplane mode because I thought the police was tracking me. That night I continued to walk down Yonge Street taking photos of everything. I remember not sleeping that night and staying a Tim Horton's waiting for the next train to come to take me out of the city. I felt as though I was being targeted by the police and therefore, I needed to leave the city. Eventually, morning came and I left the city for Niagara Falls to meet my friend Norm. While on the Go train, I started to post that I had left the city and they could not catch me. I posted that I would sue the police for harassment and the Fairmont Royal York for discrimination.

All I thought I was trying to do was promote my city and my prospective show by posting various photos on Instagram. However, what I could not see is that my posts were bizarre and too frequent. It was almost like spam. While in Niagara Falls, I felt peace and was happy to be there. I walked around Clifton Hills and along the falls to get some clarity. I met with Norman but wasn't allowed to stay at his place this time so I decided to go back to Toronto.

By the time I arrived in Toronto, it was very late, so I decided I would go to my mother's house. I arrived there around 2:30 am in the morning. My brother was staying there so he let me in and I went to sleep on the sofa. The next morning, I was in for a surprise. I woke up and started posting online immediately and was told that I was not doing well by both my mother and brother. They said I needed to stop posting online and get some help. I told them that they didn't have my insight. I called my mother Jezebel and reminded my brother that he was addicted to crack last year and need not judge me. I was hitting them below the belt but then the police arrived. They spoke to me about going to the hospital because I was unwell. I felt betrayed and started to curse at my mother and brother. They were traitors. The police took me to the local hospital and I was transferred to the William Osler Hospital on May 20, 2014.

I could not believe that my family had turned on me. I only came to the house for a little while as a stopover. Meanwhile, while they called the police on me to take me to the hospital. Wow, what a betrayal. For the next two days, I would call everyone I could think of in hopes of being released or getting help to be released.

What was so difficult was that they took away my music from me. Prior to being hospitalized, I was playing the songs **Get Lucky** by Daft Punk featuring Pharrell and Nile Rodgers and **Happy** by Pharrell on constant replay. The song **Get Lucky** was a sexual song but I took it as meaning that it was my time to get lucky and be blessed. I believed it was my time to be rich. I was going to be a millionaire and it was the right time. However, being in the hospital, I was separated from my music. There was no TV that I could listen to music on. It was simply silence and I could not take it any longer. While being in the hospital, I was forced to wear the hospital coat and I did not have a comb to do my hair. Neither did I have shampoo to wash my hair. So, to compromise, I used the bathroom soap and water to wash my hair and a pencil to comb my hair into an up do. To me this was degrading. However, I had to do what I could to make it in the hospital. The following day, I felt like the nurses ganged up on me because they forced me to take my medication by injection. I cried because I felt as though my rights were taken away from. Why were doctors and nurses able to force me to take medication that I did not want to take? Didn't I have rights? Don't I get to decide what I put in my body? How could they do this me?

Prior to being in the hospitalized, I had visited various hotels and made reservations. I would also use the washroom in each hotel. My belief was that by using the washroom I would be planting my seed in the hotel and one day I would own it. At that time, I was of the belief that I was going to be blessed like Abraham in the bible. Abraham was told that wherever he put his foot, he would gain favour and inheritance. So, I believed that wherever I went, I would receive favour. By using the washroom and making a reservation, I would be gaining favour. I had made reservations at the Marriott, Park Hyatt, Hilton, Eaton Chelsea and The Fairmont Royal York. When I made these reservations, I had no idea where the money was going to come from to pay to stay at these hotels. However, I was very confident that I would have the money because I was about to be a millionaire. Since I was hospitalized, I knew that I had to cancel all of these reservations. I contacted each hotel and cancelled the reservation. I also called many people letting them know that I was in the hospital. A few of them answered their phones and told me they would visit me. While in the hospital, I had visits from the following individuals; Amal, Budoor and Andrew from school and Minister McHugh, Chanel and Shannakay from church. This made me feel very special. They also brought me fruit. I was dying for some fruit to eat. Unfortunately in the hospital they don't give you many fruits. They give you plenty of bread though. This was frustrating. The hours and days seem to drag on forever.

While I was in the hospital I met a patient named Kendra whose room number was 41. This made me think that it was prophetic because Pharrell was 41 at the time. I therefore, believed that Kendra must be a prophet just like Pharrell. I spent a lot of time with Kendra walking the halls and telling her how special she was. She was going to be famous I told her. She asked me how I knew it, I told her I was a prophet and she believed me.

I was also fascinated with shapes. The triangle represented the illuminati. The square had 4 sides and the number 4 represented harmony. The circle represented eternity and hence Jesus. If I saw these shapes anywhere, I determined if that represented good or evil. Prior to going into the hospital, I saw many triangles and therefore concluded the illuminati had placed its mark on society. I even thought that because most houses' roofs were in a triangle, the illuminati's evil forces were surrounding the house.

Another thing I did as the prophet of the hospital was create a list of doctors and nurses that were either blessed or cursed. I determined who was blessed or cursed depending on how they treated me. On this list, they would either get a compliment or a complaint. I was going to complain to the Nurses Association and the College of Surgeons and Physicians. The doctors I was going to complain about were Dr. Hussein, Dr. Birdie and Dr. Pat from 2012. I also created a list of nurses to complain about. It was now Friday May 23, 2014, which was officially 72 hours since I had been hospitalized and I was still in the hospital. My doctor, Dr. Birdie decided not to come to work today. Instead, Dr. Hussein came instead. When he entered the room, he did not assess me but was prejudice towards me. I determined that this jerk made his decision before he entered the room. Apparently he and Dr. Birdie were in cahoots. Dr. Birdie probably told Dr. Hussein not to release me. This was nuts. Despite what I said, he was going to lock me up

Due to my reaction, he got the nurse to drug me with more medication. The following day, I woke up saddened that I was still here and wasn't released. I started to think how in one moment, one's life could change so drastically due to a label of bipolar or schizophrenia. Despite, who I was as a person, it did not matter. The label is all they saw and this saddened me.

One evening in particular at 6:41pm I started to cry. All the people I started to relate with at the hospital went home. I was all alone, so I cried. I tried to call many people so I could speak to someone and I could not get anyone. I felt as though I have blessed my friends with prayer, the word, a potential job and encouragement and they all left. As I wrote in my journal, I knew it was the devil that wanted me to feel alone. However, this caused the tears to flow much more.

I finally reached my friend Robert. I asked him if he would come and visit me. He said maybe tomorrow but he did pray for me. I was thankful but once I finished talking, in came Minister McHugh. I considered him to be a prophet. I was overjoyed that he did not forget about me. Once he left, my church sister Nyarai came. "*God is so good,*" I said to myself. Then, 30 minutes later, I get a call from my Sis Aisha saying that she was running late. I didn't expect this call but I was overjoyed because I felt as though God was answering my prayers. While we spoke on the phone, she said she would be bringing a CD and a CD player. I was overjoyed because finally, I was getting the chance to listen to music. I started to thank Jesus for this. By 6:58 pm, Sis Aisha came through and brought the Declare Jesus CD. This was a CD that was produced and performed by my church choir, APC Ministries. I could not believe how excited I was to hear music. This all happened within 17 minutes.

At that time in my life, I could not live without music. It was my lifeline. When she arrived, I instantly played a song on the CD and felt a sense of peace over my soul. I considered the hospital as a demonic place and by playing the music it might drive out those demonic spirits.

By 11:35 pm that night, I started to write in my journal again because I could not sleep. These beds were so uncomfortable. I missed my queen-sized bed. I decided that I would go to the TV room to watch some TV and hopefully fall asleep. Nurse Jas once again was getting on my nerves. When she was doing her rounds, she found me lying on the sofa and told me very harshly, *"you're not allowed to watch TV, so go to bed."* I explained if I watch some TV, it may help me to sleep. She didn't care. I decided that I would report her. I believed she was being prejudice and racist towards me. These nurses were starting to get on my nerves. I understood there were rules but I felt as though these nurses lacked compassion.

Early the following morning, I started to remember that today was supposed to be the day that I hosted my dinner for my church friends. However, unfortunately, it had to be cancelled because I was in the hospital. While in the hospital, I started to reflect and think that being here was two-fold: victory and pain. It was painful because of how the nurses, doctors and security guards treated me. They treated me like a nigger and ignorant bipolar woman. They judged me by my appearance. It was now approximately 4:10 am. I decided to ask for a cup of tea because my stomach was hurting. They told me it was too early and they didn't have any way of making it. This response gave me one more reason to hate this hospital the more. I grabbed my journal and started to write again. I wrote that the William Osler Hospital, Etobicoke site, though a hospital in name, lacked good customer service and lacked common courtesy. For example, my stomach was hurting and they told me they could not offer food or liquids while on duty for the night shift. I found that 90% of the nurses who worked for the night shift were rude, lazy, threatening, or just plain cranky. This is not the first time I observed this in a mental hospital. As far as I was concerned, all these nurses wanted to do was fraternize and make money. This made me sick. At this point, I just wanted to go home.

The following day, on Monday May 26, 2014, I was released. I decided to visit KHEM church for bible study with Bobby Somers, as I was desperate for the word of God.

Chapter 8:
Lean on Me

Though I was released from the hospital, I was still manic. I was able to convince the hospital that I could be released. Once, I was released, I continued to post online. This time, the posts were surrounding a man that was running for office with the NDP party. I started to make various videos of me freestyling and I went to the campaign office of said nominee looking to help out. I was not focused; I was all over the place. I thought that the posts I made online about him would help his campaign. However, I did not realize that my posts, when I look back on it were pretty bizarre. However, despite this, I continued to post.

I started to plan for my TV show. It was supposed to be a dinner hosted at the Gospel Café. It would start off as dinner talk and then end in some music therapy. The show was going to be recorded and produced by Daystar Media Group on June 3, 2014. I was so excited. Despite what people thought of me and my posts, I was going to meet my goal. I chose this date as a way to remember my sister Aleisha. She passed away 7 years ago on June 2 at the time. I did the taping and it was a cast of 10 people. It was supposed to be a cast of 8 but 2 additional young women showed up. Despite, this, I decided to include them. Since it was a Tuesday, the Gospel Café had a sale on wings and fried dumpling. We ordered a platter and started taping the show. The conversation was really good. Then, we ended it by having me singing the song **Happy** by Pharrell with the cast dancing in the background. We had a great time.

Now that the show had been taped, I started to get back to my routine of going to my laughing like crazy class. While in the hospital, I missed one class but got some more material because of my experience. This class gave me so much joy as I got to gain perspective on my mental illness. It also helped me to laugh at myself and not allow my illness to keep me down. After months of preparing, I finally got the chance to perform my set. It was a set of about 14 jokes and the room had about 200-300 attendees. It was held at the YMCA on Grosvenor and Yonge St. downtown. I was both excited and nervous. Finally, it was my turn to perform and I felt like I was in my element. I had so much confidence. Joke after joke, the crowd laughed more and more. This made me feel more comfortable. All in all, it was a great set. I talked about my family, my Jamaican culture and their views on mental illness, my experiences in the hospital and prison and so much more. It was great. I remember telling them about how I left shit in the slot where my food was delivered as a present for the guards while in prison. They couldn't stop laughing. Another thing that was getting back to normal was school.

Despite my illness, I came back to school in my mental health program and my school friends and teachers were so supportive. Since everything was getting back to normal, I started to re-focus on creating my talk show to raise awareness for mental illness. In an effort to gain support, I contacted my Member of Parliament, Rathika, to arrange a meeting. I was eventually granted a meeting. I shared my talk show idea with her and asked for her support. She was in full support of the idea. We did an interview with my iPad and took photos to be posted online. She also agreed to write a letter of support for the talk show to help me as I raised money for it. In addition, she agreed to be my mentor. Considering what had happened a few months back, I felt really good that my life was getting back to normal.

In order to promote my talk show, I asked one of the church brothers to help me by doing a promotional video of me. I shared my testimony of being bipolar and almost jumping over the bridge. It was a moving testimony. To complete the video, the church brother took some great photos of me to be used in my promotional material and my website. It looked really good. I had promoted this so much, that I was able to recruit a few additional people from church as cast of the show. Sadly, the two young men I met a few months back were too busy to be cast members on the show, so, I revised it. Slowly, my reputation was being rebuilt and my life had meaning. The idea of the show was growing. I had a website and started raising money online. I shared the idea with my pastor and he loved it also. I asked for permission to share the idea with the church and he said yes. I did the presentation and after received donations of over $400 to start. Other members told me they would donate at a later date and they did. Many people told me how proud they were of me and wished me many blessings. After doing various interviews with many different people in the community, my pastor did an interview with me. He shared both a practical and spiritual perspective on mental health. We talked about demons and mental illness and other issues. In the end we had about 1000 views. Of all my videos, this one received the most views.

The following month, I returned back to school in the TPE program and was asked to do an interview by the school newspaper, The Dialog at George Brown College. I was really excited to do this interview. I talked about the show and how I was using my mental illness to make an impact and they loved it. They loved it so much that they decided to feature me on the cover of the newspaper. I was stoked! This was my first cover story ever. My face was featured in all three campuses for two whole weeks. I picked up copies for all my friends and family. I was so proud of my accomplishment. God was really doing a mighty work in my life.

I was truly happy; I was in my last semester for the TPE program and getting so much positive feedback. To continue promoting the show, I continued to do interviews. I did interviews with 4 classmates living with mental illness, Tiffany Ford (TDSB trustee nominee at the time), another Pastor, the leaders of Movember, Dewitt Lee and Dr. Benjamin Goldstein from Sunnybrook Hospital. In total, I did 20 videos over the span of 4 months. Due to this new format, we decided that we would re-tape the show, as its new focus was mental health. Melica from Daystar Media Group, my producer at the time and I worked on setting up a new video shoot date. It was set for the first week of December 2014.

In order to further promote the show, I was given the opportunity to be a guest on CHRY 105.5 radio at York University. This was my first time on radio so I made sure that I taped it for my records. I was hilarious and the show did really well. As the days approached, I was so focused on getting my show up and raising money, that I did not notice that I was becoming manic. My posts online had increased. My mood was elevated but I was determined to record the show. I was not going to allow my illness to stop my progress. I had worked my butt off. My family started to express their concern but all I cared about was the show.

Finally, the day came and we recorded. Sadly, not all the cast members showed up and we had to add a few people as cast members who showed up to support. I shared my testimony and people asked me questions, and it was great. Once it was done, I took a sigh of relief. I did it. The next goal was to raise the rest of money to get the show to be aired on YES TV. Over the past few months, I had been in contact with the network's representative in charge of the television shows that were on the roster. We had decided that we would do a pilot and I would pay for one episode. This would cost me under $500. I was so excited. All I had to do was raise a few more dollars and get the show edited for TV. I was so close. Over the Christmas holiday, my assistant, Gaysha and I contacted at least 25 friends and family members trying to raise the money. We were able to raise the money and I was thankful.

In the New Year, January 2015, the edited version comes back to me and the audio is too low. You could barely hear anyone except me because I naturally have a loud voice. However, the other cast members were difficult to hear. Despite, this, we decided to the send the copy to YES TV in hopes that they could air it. Sadly, they said we would either have to re-edit it or re-tape it. I was heartbroken but I knew what needed to be done. So, I spoke with Melica and told her that we needed to redo it. She agreed and said she wouldn't charge extra since the error was on her end. The new date of the television show was January 20th, 2015. If we had re-taped it on the 20th, we would be able to have the show aired in February. This was how I promoted it to everyone. I told them that their donations would pay for the airing of our show in February. Friends and family were excited about it. However, my mother was concerned about me. I personally felt like my mother was jealous of me. I did not know why she was trying to stop me.

Exactly one day before we were going to tape the show, my mother had the police come to my home and instructed to take me to the mental hospital. I was livid. She did it again. She is trying to stop me. I was only one day away from taping the show again. I thought, *"Why would she do this to me?"* I was sent to CAMH for two weeks. I was pissed. Am I cursed? Why does stuff like this always happen as I am close to succeeding? I did not understand.

I stayed in CAMH and finally was able to prove to them that I was sane enough to go home, so I was released. Considering how close I was to having my show on television, led me to feel like a failure. How will I start again?

As the days passed, my mood became more and more dark. I started to think about dying. I started to fantasize about getting a gun. Where would I go? How would I get one? I stopped myself as I realized that I was suicidal. I decided on Friday February 6, 2015, that I would check myself into CAMH again. Unlike other times, I chose to go to the hospital. I needed help. As I approached the hospital, I took out my iPhone and took a photo of myself in front of CAMH. I used that photo to post on Instagram and Facebook with a caption that expressed that I was going to the hospital because I was suicidal. Once done, I entered the building to be assessed. I remember feeling nervous as I sat in the lobby waiting to be called into the secured waiting area. Finally, they called me in and the door locks behind me. Once you are in the waiting room, you never know what you are going to see. Also, the door is locked to prevent you from leaving without their permission, should you try to escape. I remember waiting in the room and there was another man in there that was erratic. He cursed and swore that he didn't belong there. He would walk back and forth becoming angrier as the moments passed. Then, he started to bang on the wall. A nurse finally came out and calmly spoke to him. She told him that he could not be released and to wait a few minutes. He became even angrier as she shut the door.

Then it was my time to go into the assessment room. I met with an intake nurse and asked me the standard questions. *"What brings in to the hospital today?"* I told her I was suicidal and needed help.

She continued, *"Have you tried to commit suicide?"* I explained that I had suicidal ideations and thought about getting a gun. I also told them that I had tried to commit suicide in the past. She asked me a few more questions and then asked me to go back to the waiting room. I waited for some time and then I was asked to come back in the private room. They told me that they were going to admit me. They put a hospital bracelet on me and led me upstairs. This time, I was sent in the General Psychiatry Unit (GPU) on the 5th floor. I recognized a few of the nurses from my last stay. Some of them were shocked to see me. However, I did not let the bother me. I waited in the common area for about 30 minutes and then was escorted to my new shared room. I was worried about who my roommate might be. You never know what you're going to get with a roommate. They could be homeless, they could steal, they could have horrible body odor, or they could be highly unstable. Thankfully, I was put into a room with a depressed older woman that later I determined was high functioning. She was very nice. I had a sigh of relief.

It was the weekend at CAMH and most of the doctors weren't available, so it was a quiet weekend. There were different types of people that were at the hospital. I made a few friends that weekend and started to chat with them. One gentleman was in his 40s, another in his 50s and my roommate in her 40s. We got to know each other and started to get along. By the time, Sunday came around, I was started to feel hopeful. While in the hospital, I came across a sign that said the word HOPE. I decided to take a selfie with me standing under it and post it to Instagram and Facebook with the caption, *"While here at the hospital, I came across this. I found it inspirational."* <u>On Friday I was hopeless, today I am hopeful. #Mentalillness #suicide #recovery #healing</u>. Though I was hospitalized, I was gaining strength. I spent the next few days either in the common area or the arts room.

Music was a very important part of my life and there was a piano. I wasn't the best piano player but I understood chords so I played the song, **"Lean on me."** I closed the door and started to belt out the song with all of my being. I felt such healing and comfort as I sang the song. Then, the door opens so I stopped singing. The gentleman at the door says to continue, as he wanted to listen as well. So I continued to sing and he started to tap is foot and move to the rhythm. It was a beautiful moment.

The next day, I met my doctor, a female. Normally, I did not like females because I felt they were haters and were threatened by me. I asked her where she was from as white doctors had traumatized me and I was done with them. She was Spanish. Since she was an immigrant, I felt comfortable with her. I told her my feelings about white people and why I no longer wanted white doctors. She said she understood. She asked me about my mood and I told her that I was still depressed, suicidal but hopeful. I just needed help. She said they would do everything to help me. I told her that my medication, lithium, had not been working and that I had a few episodes while taking it. She was shocked as this medication worked for many people. However, she decided to try me on two new prescriptions effective immediately. After a few days, I started to notice a different. My mood was improving.

While at the hospital, I had a few visitors and this made me happy. One particular visit was my friends from school, Budoor, Heather and Chantal. I was so happy to see them. They also brought fruit, chips and cookies. These ladies were awesome. They will never know how much I appreciated their visit. While at the hospital, my birthday passed and I was a bit depressed that I was spending it in the hospital. I should have been spending it with friends, laughing and having a great time. However, I had been in a hospital dealing with depression. While in the hospital, one of the residents recognized it was my birthday and gave me a flower. Where they got said flower, I do not know. I was truly grateful.

There were a few things in the common room. There was the TV, the chairs and table for lunch, books, games and two computers. I decided to go onto to the computer to see my birthday wishes. I was so shocked on how many people wished me a happy birthday. I received 59 birthday wishes. This made me smile. The following day, I wrote a quick post on my Facebook wall: *"I would like to thank everyone who took the time to say happy birthday to me on my Facebook timeline. Unlike other years, it had a much more special meaning for me. Being in the hospital has been a bit difficult but when you see that there are some people who still care about you, it means a lot. Some people they may disregard those simple words posted on their timeline but for me, it was a small reminder that people still loved me and cared for me. Thank you for this reminder. #VirtualHug.*

I was truly thankful and blessed to have these individuals in my life and thankful that I lived to see another year. I was committed to make sure that the next birthday would be different.

It had been a week and a half since I was admitted into the hospital. I was improving and my doctor finally decided that I could get a day pass to go out. While outside on Wednesday February 18, 2015, I decided that I would visit the Queen Street site of CAMH because I had just accepted to attend a program called AIM (Anxiety and Mood Disorders). This program was an in-patient program where the residents would live there for 28 days. I decided I would check out the campus and see what I thought. I went into the building and asked for a tour. I told them that I would going to the site next month and wanted to see what it was like. Once again, it was on a locked floor. Only the receptionist or nurse could open the door. The rooms were extremely tiny but they were private. They had a common area and the kitchen was open. It was nice. Once I was done my tour I left the building and continued to walk outside until I discovered this beautiful mural that said the words in large caps YOU'VE CHANGED. I was so thankful and hopeful. I told myself, *"Yes, one day, these words will be true for me."* This was my goal; I wanted my illness to no longer enslave me. Instead, I would be master of my disease. I planned on managing my disease and my relationships. With that said, I decided to post it on my Facebook wall and Instagram.

On February 20, 2015, I was finally released from the hospital. Apparently, you had to be out of the hospital for at least two weeks before you can get into the program. I was given a two weeks supply of my medication and a prescription from my doctor. When I came out, though no longer depressed, my mood was elevated. I thought I was simply happy but when I think about it and I look back on my Facebook timeline, I realize I was manic. Once again, I created a new business. I was going to start a consulting business where I would provide consulting in life, business and mental health. For this business, I would charge $144 per hour with a $70 non-refundable deposit. I also was bold enough to mention how my time was precious and I thought it was time I receive pay for the energy that I was exerting. I tagged almost 53 people in this post. The next post I made was about going back to school to study music at Spelman College in Atlanta, Georgia. I talked about multiple intelligences and that I was overlooked because most schools only consider audio and visual intelligences. I felt like my musical and mathematical intelligences would consider me a genius. This is what I thought of myself. I was a genius. I wanted the world to know that I was a genius and started to post again. Some of the consistent things that were in my collages were my IAMCLEONI banner and four flags representing the countries my businesses would be located in. The four countries were as follows: Jamaica, United Kingdom, USA and Canada.

I also posted about Stevie Wonder. While in the hospital, I played a lot of Stevie Wonder in the music and arts room. My posts were based on the different places I had been. I had been to Queen's Park, city hall, and various subway stations. The next thing I would post about is Pharrell. He was a King and Prophet in my book.

One night while unpacking and thinking about the AIM program, I had a thought that if I stayed in Toronto, the city was going to destroy me. I decided I was no longer going to the program. In fear, I packed my bag and left town. I decided that I needed to see my mentor Member of Parliament Rathika in Ottawa. So, I got on the bus and went to Ottawa to see her. I did not have a place to stay so I stayed in a shelter. However, to get Wi-Fi while in Ottawa, I went to different hotels like the Westin and the Marriott. When I arrived, I went to Parliament to see MP Rathika but there was a flood in the building and her staff was back in Toronto. I was devastated. I came all this way and she wasn't there. I decided to see my other friend in politics, Judy Sgro. Judy's office is across the street from the Supreme Court of Canada in the Justice building. I went in and met with her executive assistant Greg. We chatted and I told him that I wanted to file lawsuits against a few doctors and wanted to know what the procedures were. He referred me to a law firm. He also gave me something to eat. He told me that I could buy anything in the store. I took food to last me for the day and thanked him.

I went on my way to check out the law firm. Unfortunately, they did not offer contingency and I would have to pay a deposit. This saddened me. While in Ottawa, I thought I was going to make Ottawa my new home because people were much nicer.

I went into the Rideau Mall and started to collect various business cards from businesses that I wanted to shop in or bless. I went to Hudson's Bay and decided that I needed a suitcase and hat for my head. I found a red suitcase that was on sale. I also found a fur hat with the dog-ears that was also on sale. I had a great day in the mall and collected various cards and wanted to bless many people. Though people were nice, I went to the mall and met a man named Trevor who was very pleasant. I went to the Apple store and was talking about buying almost $10,000 in goods. However, I believed I would have the money because of my new business. So in my mind I was pre-shopping. However, one of the black managers came to me while speaking to Tyler the representative and said that I overspent my welcome. I left the store and suddenly went on my knees and shouted, *"This is a protest! This manager treated me like a nigger and I want everyone to know."* I guess I cracked. They contacted the security and when I saw them coming, I started to leave the mall. They kept calling me and I kept shouting in the mall, *"They treated me like a nigger. I am a not a nigger. You are all racists."* Finally, I left the mall and I heard them shouting, *"You are not welcome here. If you return, we will call the police."* I gave them the finger and left.

While in Ottawa, I had been posting threatening posts about the Parliament. I wished death upon Stephen Harper, the prime minister at the time, and every racist politician except MP Rathika and MP Judy. I had also posted that I was going to sue the government for treating me like a nigger. I wanted to sue them for $17.8 million dollars for their treatment. If they didn't pay, I would sue for $144 million. I also offered a job to an online comedian for an obscene amount of money, $88,888 to be exact. This money would be paid from my settlement from the government. I would continue to post various photos of me cursing the Parliament. I would do this because I thought I was a prophet and hence had the right to wish a curse on them. I believed that my job as a global prophet was to bless and curse people, institutions, and governments. Therefore, in my mind, I wasn't doing anything wrong. After cursing Parliament, I decided to go back to the shelter I had been staying at.

As I arrived back in the shelter, I received a call from the Ottawa police. They said that they had been following my Twitter and Facebook account and were concerned about my posts. They wanted to speak to me. They asked me if I was still staying at the shelter. My eyes widened. How did they know? Then, I remembered, I had posted my location earlier this morning before I left. So, they asked if I could meet with them. They asked me if I knew that the posts I was posting could be seen as a terror attack on the government. I was shocked as I thought I was just expressing my freedom of speech. However, they did not think so. They wanted to meet me, so I told them that they could come. As soon as I hung up the phone, I realized that I needed to get out of Ottawa a.s.a.p. and go to Montreal. In a hurry, I packed up my bags and left the shelter for the VIA rail train station. While enroute, I turned off my data and acted as though I did nothing wrong. I was scared. I did not want to get caught. While at the bus station, I was fearful and knew I needed to get out of Ottawa as soon as possible. I purchased my ticket and waited for my bus. While in the bus station, I noticed the police, so I put on my new fur hat and acted like everything was normal. Thankfully, my bus arrived and I boarded it. Sayonara Ottawa, Montreal here I come.

Chapter 9:
Virtual Insanity

I was relieved that I made it to Montreal with no problems. I searched for a hostel to stay in to save money. I found one and it was really nice. The next morning at breakfast, I met all these backpackers from France. They were very cool, so we took photos together for Instagram and I posted the location. Then, I decided that I would go for a walk. Next thing I noticed, that the Montreal Police was directly behind my hostel. I did not think anything of it. So, I continued to walk and then, as I was about to walk back, I noticed police officers coming out of my hostel. I knew they were looking for me. Though terrified, I kept my cool and walked and turned up my music and started to sing. I walked pass the officer singing. I smiled at him. He returned the smile. Then, when I saw them go back into their car and drive away, I went back into my hostel and told myself that it was time to leave. I packed up my bag and went into the washroom to look up tickets to go to Nova Scotia. I told myself that I wanted to go there because this was where the original black slaves came. I believed that by being there I wouldn't experience as much racism as I had experienced. I got my ticket and noted the bus station location.

As I was about to leave the hostel, I noticed there was a blockade of police officers blocking the street. I was worried and started to believe they were looking for me. So, to avoid it, I called a taxi and asked the driver to take me to a mall. I figured I would walk around and then go to the bus station. As usual, I took many selfies of myself in front of stores that I deemed blessed. I also, requested business cards from stores I found favourable. I told myself that one day when I get my millions, I would return and shop there. I continued to travel across the city until it was time for me to catch my bus. I went to the bus station and bid Montreal adieu.

    I was so excited to go to Nova Scotia; I learned so much about this province from my history classes while studying at the University of Toronto. I learned that Nova Scotia was a place where many Black slaves from the United States called home when escaping. It was home to Loyalists, Maroons, Caribbean's, and refugees among others. I knew that this would become my new home. In order to get to Nova Scotia, we first crossed the border from Quebec into New Brunswick. Upon arriving in New Brunswick, I was told that I would have to wait a few hours for the next bus to Nova Scotia. I was a bit frustrated but took the opportunity to do some site seeing as I had never been to this province.

    The first thing I discovered was a hotel. I went in and asked the concierge to see their boardrooms. My plan was to come back here and host my first executive meeting in New Brunswick. However, once again, there was a missing factor, money! That did not matter to me because I believed that I was going to win a large settlement through my lawsuits. After checking out the boardrooms, I told the representative that I would be back in a few weeks and would book the boardroom for 13 people. Once done, I decided to walk through the city but unfortunately it started to rain. As I walked, I discovered a law firm and decided to go in. In my eyes, I would get a lawyer from a different province than my home and use them to file my lawsuits with them. I took a business card and left. When I left the building and continued to walk, I discovered a dinner theatre restaurant and decided to go in. I received a tour of the place and asked about their reservations process. They told me about the process and I told them that I would be back to book it for a party.

Meanwhile, since I left Ontario, the fraud department thought that someone was using my credit card and put a block on it. I had to go to a branch of my bank that was open. I finally found one and told them about my predicament. They gave me a new card and dispensed the money I requested. Once I was done at the bank, I checked the time and realized that it was almost time for my bus to come. I started to panic; as there was no way that I could walk back in time. So, I started to look for a cab as I quickly walked back. Frantically, I would back and forth in search of a cab. If I missed this bus, I might get stuck in this province with no money or place to go.

Thankfully a cab came out of nowhere and stopped for me. *"Excuse me sir, but I'm running late and might miss my bus, can you go as quickly as possible?"* He responded, *"I'll do the best I can."* While riding in the car, I started to tell him more about myself and asked him about the province. He told me that it was a family city and province. I told him I was going to Nova Scotia and he immediately told me that I would enjoy myself there in comparison. He said that New Brunswick is a boring province. I believed him and then we arrived. My bus was already there waiting for the passengers to board the bus. If I had not taken the cab, I would have missed my bus and been stranded. I boarded the bus and to Nova

Scotia I went. I slept most of the way but woke up when we arrived in Halifax. I knew I was home. There was something in the air. The bus conductor finally made his announcement that we had arrived in Halifax, Nova Scotia and we could leave the bus and pick up our luggage. I got off the bus, picked up my luggage and smelled the winter air. Now, it was time to find a place to stay. After searching on the Internet, I found a shelter in Halifax. It was in a nice little house called The Barry House. I met the intake worker and she asked me various questions. I answered them and they gave me my own room. I later discovered that they gave me my own room because they were concerned about my mental state but still allowed me in.

As usual, I went on social media and made a video about it. I posted that they gave me a room to myself because they think I'm crazy and I was proud of it. I was really thankful to have my own room because I didn't want stuff like my tripod to get stolen. To make myself more comfortable, I unpacked my luggage into the drawers. Once done, I went downstairs to get something to eat, as I was really hungry. The ladies were really nice. I met one young lady in particular that was really young, about the age of my deceased sister Aleisha. She was native with a shaved head. I took a photo with her and said that she would be perfect for being a business partner. You see, everywhere I went, I was always scouting for new business partners. It all depended on the energy of the person. Though this young lady had a checkered past, I thought she represented the missing link to my business, a native person. I was so thankful to have met her.

The next morning, I left the shelter to go site seeing. I walked everywhere and took many photos. I remember getting to Global TV Nova Scotia. I made a video in front of the station saying, if

Global TV was interested in interviewing me about my trials, they could contact me. I tagged them and many others in the post on Instagram. After posting, I continued to walk and post on Instagram in my new account @theisraelite88. While there, I found the local CMHA (Canadian Mental Health Association) of Halifax and decided to go in. I took various brochures and asked about their programs and support groups. I told them about my TV show and they were excited as well. The card said there were two locations in Nova Scotia; the second location was in Dartmouth, which was just across the bridge.

I decided to walk across the bridge and discovered Dartmouth. Dartmouth was quieter than Halifax and was by the water. After walking around the city, I decided that when I buy my house, I would look for a place in Dartmouth. To show that I was serious, I made an appointment with Scotiabank in Dartmouth to open a bank account. After that, I posted a photo that showed the card from CMHA and my current shelter. That was a mistake!

Despite this, I continued to travel and take photos of various landmarks and myself. I visited the main library, the black business association, the mall, and Dalhousie University.

I stayed at the Barry House for about 3 days and then it happened. I was called down to the office at my shelter. They told me to come with my suitcases packed. I packed everything up and then went downstairs. With no explanation, they asked me to leave. I was pissed. I let them know about it. I called them racist bitches and told them that I would sue them for their discrimination. I took photos and said that I would post their faces on Instagram and would f**k them up. I left the building and walked around the city with my suitcase for hours. I was worried. Where would I stay now?

I had no money. After hours of walking, the sun started to set and it was now evening. I determined that I would find a Tim Horton's and stay there until I found another shelter. However, I did not know where I was going. I found this gentleman and asked him where it was. He told me to go down this path and I would find it. I travelled along the path and I ended up getting deeper and deeper into the woods. I was truly lost.

I had to keep walking and needed to get out of this forest. It had now been about four hours of walking in the snow with my suitcase at night. I started to pray and then I became really tired. I decided that I would lie down in the snow and take a nap. I started to cry because I was lost, cold and tired. There it was I was homeless and laying in the snow. I slept for about 15 minutes and then received a sudden burst of energy. I had the strength to keep walking. I walked until I saw the highway. I knew that if I kept walking, I would find something. I walked for another two hours and then, there it was a hotel. I went inside and asked if I could get warm for a bit because I was lost. He said it was fine. Then, suddenly, I fainted and had a seizure in the hotel. The attendant called the ambulance as I had multiple seizures. The ambulance finally arrived around 2:30am. I stopped seizing but was taken to the Dartmouth General Hospital.

While in the hospital, I started to get warm. I wanted to see the doctor and get released. They told me I would see a doctor very soon so I fell asleep and two hours later, still no doctor. I went over to the nurses and asked when I would see a doctor to only find them laughing and joking around. They said, I would see a doctor soon and I was frustrated. I went back to my room and was thinking, *"These people are trying to have me committed."*

I decided to put on my clothing and leave the hospital. They sent a security officer after me. He kept calling me and I kept telling him to f**k off. He followed me and continued to yell at me to come back. I kept walking and then finally I was off the grounds and he turned back. Though I had left the hospital, I did not know where I was going. However, I started to pray and ask God to lead me. So, I walked through different neighbourhoods and finally after 3 hours of walking, I found a bus stop. I asked the bus driver for a lift as I told him I was lost. He said it was fine and took me to a mall in Halifax. It was about 9am on March 8, 2015 and I went into the mall. While there, I turned on my data and took photos. I went upstairs to an employment centre to make a phone call to find a new shelter.

Next thing I know, the police met me there. I asked them what they wanted. *"We were advised that the hospital put a form 1 on you and said you left the hospital. We are here to take you to the hospital."* I was pissed.

I arrived at the Abbie J. Lane Mental Hospital on March 8, 2015 and was surprisedly thankful because Nova Scotia felt like home. While at the hospital, I met this really cool Caucasian lady named Nancy and we clicked immediately. We talked about everything and it was good. Since I started to feel like Nova Scotia was home, I decided to post on social media once again. This time I posted an angry post letting all my Ontario friends and enemies know that I was home and currently staying in the psychiatric ward. I wanted everyone to know that I was leaving Ontario for good and that I was going to make Nova Scotia my new home. I was sick and tired of the abuse I experienced in Ontario. I wanted everyone I knew in Ontario to know that I had given 33 years of life to Ontario and I had enough. I wanted a fresh start. Even though I was in the mental ward, I felt peace. I felt like I was finally going to get treated for the problems that I had.

I really felt that I was misdiagnosed with Bipolar and that I had PTSD. I felt like I went through a lot of trauma and was dealing with the stress of it all. I just wanted to be understood and here in Nova Scotia, the doctors were actually considering if I indeed had PTSD; that made me feel good.

My first doctor was a white female and she seemed nice at first but eventually I started to feel judged by her. When I was back in Toronto, I started to grow distrust to all white people including white females who I felt were intimidated by my intelligence. So when I met my new doctor who was a white female, I was very hesitant. Thought hesitant, due to her friendly demeanor, I thought I would give her a chance. We met in the meeting room with another white nursing student. I was very concerned but thought it would not be that bad. She asked me questions about what I was doing in Nova Scotia and why I thought I was here. I told her my story of leaving Toronto and that I just wanted to make Nova Scotia my new home. I told her some of my plans and that I had distrust for white people due to how I had been treated. She reminded me that she was white. I told her that I was giving her a chance and she smiled. I told her that while in Nova Scotia, I wanted to be treated for PTSD.

However, after assessing me, she told me that she did not believe I had PTSD and only showed signs of being Bipolar. When she said that, I snapped and said, *"I knew this was about to be some bullshit! I knew you white people wouldn't listen to me. I knew you would be quick to call me bipolar. F**k this. I want a black doctor. I am tired of you white people. Are we done here?"* She replied, *"You seem irritable, I think we should give you something to calm you down."* I responded, *"You cannot force me to take medication. I want a second opinion, and I want a black doctor."* Shortly after this discussion, which now turned into a heated argument, I left the room and went back into the common areas. Moments later one of the nurses on duty came to me with two security officers and medication to calm me down. They gave me two options: either take the pill voluntarily or by force. I chose to take the pill voluntarily.

Due to how I felt this doctor treated me, I decided to file a complaint and request a black doctor. I refused to cooperate with white people anymore because they were racist in my books. My complaint made its way to the executive doctors and I was granted my wish. I was given a new doctor, a black African doctor. I had my first meeting with him where I told him how much I appreciated having a black doctor. He smiled but informed that his colleagues were just as good. I then proceeded to tell my story and how racist people of authority had treated me. I told him my plans for my new business and that I wanted to go back to school to study music and sing for the armed forces. I also told him that I wanted to be treated for PTSD. Sadly, this doctor was no different. He then told me that my mother called the hospital and wanted to speak with me. I was furious with my mother. I thought she was being influenced by the devil. I thought a spirit called Jezebel was influencing her. I considered myself to be a prophet that was being persecuted by the spirit of Jezebel. My mother just so happened to be one of the many Jezebels I had encountered since I began my journey. So, when the doctor said she wanted to talk to me, I was upset. (She had called the hospital a few times earlier and I refused her calls each time.) I repeated to the doctor that I did not want to speak to her. However, this doctor said I should reconsider my decision. I left the meeting feeling as though I was not being listened to. I felt like the doctor was a sexist African male influenced by his culture, which said women were to be silent rather than great. In my eyes, he was another enemy.

While in the hospital, I started to listen to my gospel music for direction. Every song had a specific meaning for me. At that time, I had an idea to start a business named #Musictherapy42. With this business, I would create different CDs that were therapy for the mind. Also, I would host dance parties in hotels in different countries in major cities. The specific artists that would be added in this CD would be people that I considered either Prophets or Apostles. For example, on March 20, 2015 at 6:00pm, it was revealed to me that Tye Tribbet who sung the song "**Good**" was an Israelite prophet. Therefore, like Pharrell, he represented another artist that I should listen to in order to receive my therapy.

It was Saturday March 21, 2015 at 6:01 am when I woke up and started to create a list of 10 songs that I called "The New Life, The New Day." I listened to these songs from 6:01 am to 7:31 am. These songs were not only gospel songs but also a few secular artists like India Arie, Jill Scott, and Stevie Wonder. At the end of the music, I added up the digits of the times that I listened to each song. When I added it up, it was 126. From this number, I deduced that I should go to Acts 1:8 because when you added 6 and 2 you get 8. When placed side by side, you get 1:8. In particular, this scripture said the following,

"But ye shall receive power after that the Holy Ghost is come upon you and ye shall be witnesses unto me both in Jerusalem, and all Judea, and in Samaria, and unto the uttermost part of the earth."

With this verse, I saw it as confirmation that I would experience a new life of power and influence. I then proceeded to write in my journal a to-do list of things that I wanted to get done while in Nova Scotia. The list went as follows:

1. Get a Nova Scotia phone number with Virgin Mobile.
2. Call my father to get him to book me a flight to Jamaica

3. Say my final goodbye to my mother.
4. Contact Melica to see if she is still interested in HappyHome42 or do I need to find someone else.
5. Contact Clinroy (my brother) to move my stuff in storage.
6. Contact Gaysha to see if she wants my apartment.
7. Contact Paladin to compliment Shian and Matthew (two security officers) and ask them to send a quote for 4 officers for my #Musictherapy42 business.

After writing this down, I decided that I would speak to my mother. The next time I saw my doctor, he asked me once again if I wanted to see my mother as she said she would be flying down to Nova Scotia to see me. I told him that I would see her to tell her my final goodbye.

In preparation for her visit, I decided I would create an agenda for our meeting. I wrote that I would start in prayer, read about Jezebel from the book of Revelations, explain my sister Aleisha's death, and explain that I discovered that Aleisha was a prophet as I was. I would go on to explain that ever since I was 13 (an illuminati number [13 bloodlines in the Illuminati]) the illuminati have been trying to kill me. Then I would decode the bottom numbers of my passport, which added up to 63, which was the year that my mother was born. I would then confront her, stating that she was a Jezebel trying to hold me back and prevent me from being a prophet. The next thing I would do is tell her to call my father and ask him to be my substitute decision maker or I would take her to court and ensure that she lost her job and her business JAAMM idol. Finally, I would say that although I love her, she is too controlling like Jezebel and that she has to apologize to my church by April 12th for her role in causing me to become sick or she would become a lunatic ten times worse than I am.

The day finally came when I was to meet my mother. I met her with my black doctor and a nursing student and I started to share the things on my agenda. I blamed her for the death of my sister because just like Jezebel sacrificed her children, I believed that my mother sacrificed my sister. I also told her that I no longer wanted anything to do with her. She responded to the doctor by saying that they were to keep me in the hospital for as long as possible as she believed that I was not doing well. I became enraged and told her I no longer wanted to see her again and that I would take her to court to have her removed as my mother. When I walked out of the room, she had this shocked look on her face but I did not care.

I left her and the doctor to speak, went back to my room and started to journal again. It was 12:54pm and I was so upset. I wrote that she would either REPENT or DIE by her birthday April 14, 2015. I turned on my music and the song that was playing was **"Virtual Insanity"** by Jamiroquai which confirmed to me that she definitely was going to become a lunatic.

After a few weeks of being locked up in the hospital, I decided that I was done. I got my jacket, packed my stuff and demanded that the nurses let me out. I believed that I was prisoner and they needed to release me. They told me to calm down. I told them to *"F**k off and let me out!"* They contacted the security. When they arrived, they told me to calm down or they would put me in isolation. I continued to shout and complain that I wanted to leave. The security proceeded to grab me and pull me into the room. I decided that I was not going down without a fight. I punched the officer in the face and tackled him to the ground. He tried to restrain me as he stood over me, so I spit in his face. The other officer, tried to hold my feet down. I started to scream and then, it was done, I was given a needle and locked in the room. I started to bang on the door and scream, *"F**k off and let me out!"* The nurses and officers continued to ignore me. Eventually, I gave up and sat down in a corner and started to cry, as I did not understand why the Lord allowed me to go through such pain. Eventually, I started to feel drowsy due to the medication, so I fell asleep.

When I eventually woke up, it turned out that I had been sleeping for at least 8 hours. I found a plate of food on the ground waiting for me. I was so hungry that I ate the food. Then, I went back to the door and started to knock on the door requesting to come out of the room. They asked me if I was going to behave and I told them yes. They finally let me out and I went to my room. I was still drowsy from the medication and since it was late, I decided to go back to bed.

Chapter 10:
Music Therapy

One morning as I was relaxing in the common room, I heard a commotion as security guards were bringing in a new patient. He was not happy to be sent to the hospital. He pulled and tugged at the security officers and yelled, *"Yo guy, let go of me!"* He continued to fight and yell. Eventually, he was put into the isolation room and the nurses came in with needles to sedate him. I didn't know why he was here but I was upset because he, like me, was black. I immediately started to think to myself, *"you see that is what they want to do to us; they want to silence us."* I continued to watch but was helpless to do anything about it. Hours, later, the gentleman calmed down and was released from the room to see his family in the common room. They tried to convince him that it was the best thing for him to be in the hospital. He was not having it. He stood by the window and argued with his family and told them he didn't belong there. Then, eventually, his family hugged him and said their goodbyes. Just a few minutes after they left the boy goes back to the window and jumps out! I screamed because I could not believe that this just happened. Thankfully, he landed on his feet and took off running. The nurses came in the room to see what the matter was. One of the patients told them that the client just jumped out the window. *"He what?"* they exclaimed. *"We need to call the police,"* they continued.

Immediately, the nurses called the security and the police to locate the escapee.

I stood there amazed and shocked that this boy would just jump out the window. I was also happy that he escaped and started to laugh at the irony of it all. I called him Spiderman. This whole scenario was hilarious to me as I started to see this young man as my hero. He escaped. They didn't succeed in holding this black man down. They failed, he won. His family frantically came back into the hospital and they were pissed. *"How could you let this happen?"* The nurses asked them to calm down and ushered them into one of the meeting rooms. I continued to find this whole ordeal hilarious. I started to talk with some of the patients about this. We prayed that he was okay but was also happy that he was able to get out of this horrible place. Sadly, hours later, they found the boy, brought him back to the hospital and put him in a new ward in isolation.

I was given the opportunity to see my doctors daily so they could assess me and see how I was doing. On one particular morning, I met with the doctors and the resident and we talked about my progress. They complimented me and told me that I was doing much better. The doctor recommended that I try a new drug called Risperidone. I asked them about the medication that was given to me in Ontario and why I couldn't take that. He dismissed my concerns and told me that this was a better drug. He then gave me a paper that had some information about it. I left the meeting with the paper and went into my room. I started to talk to my roommate about the new drug they wanted to give me. She highly recommended against it. She told me some of her horror stories and the side effects. I started to worry.

The following day, I went back to the doctor and told him my concerns. He once again dismissed my concerns but told me that those side effects were rare and that this was a good drug. Because I wanted to get out soon, I decided to take the drug.

My condition continued to improve and I was getting along with the nurses and security officers. Due to this, when I met with my doctor for my regular assessment, I decided to ask him for a day pass to be able to leave the premises. He took a day to think about and then approved me. I was so thankful and glad to be able to leave the hospital even for just a few hours. The day I was given my pass, I was given a pass for two hours. I took the day to take a walk around the community. It was really cold but I did not care. I was outside. I was able to feel the sun on my face. I was free, even if it was just for a few hours. Since they allowed me to have my phone, I was able to listen to my music. I would sing on the top of my lungs and dance in the snow. People stared but I did not care. They did not know my situation. I was full of joy. My time was almost up so I went back to the hospital. The nurses asked me if I enjoyed my pass. I told them that I did. From that day on, I would continue to get passes and I would use them to do different things such as go to the library, take a walk, or do some planning for my new business. Things were looking up.

A week had passed and the length of my passes went up to 6 hours. I still did not get to the point where I could get to stay out overnight but I was thankful for the 6 hours, as it was a lot of time.

One day on my pass, I decided to use the pass to visit a hotel and request to see their ballroom. I checked it out and made a video of me at the hotel. I told the representative that I wanted to host a dinner there for my new business and talk show. They were excited. Funny thing that they did not know was that I had no money to plan this event. However, in my mind, the money would come. I would sell tickets and that is how I would pay for the venue. Despite not having money, I asked them to send me a contract and I would let them know when I had the deposit. We shook hands and I left the hotel and went back to the hospital.

    Another day, I took my 6-hour pass to go downtown. I went everywhere. I took pictures wherever I went but I did not post them online because I was concerned that the police would follow me again. Once I was done my walk, I went back to the hospital. Each time I came back to the hospital, I felt so refreshed because if only for a few hours, I could be a human being. I was not locked up or caged in a stuffy hospital.

    Approximately a week later, just a few days before Good Friday, I decided to request an overnight pass so I could go to church. For Christians, Good Friday and Easter were second to Christmas. It was so important that I be allowed to go to church. If I was given the chance to get the overnight pass, I would have been able to stay with a church member. I made all the plans and was prepared with all the details to show my doctor to get approval. I met with my doctor and explained that I wanted to go to the Good Friday service and Easter Sunday service and requested a weekend pass. Despite how prepared I was and my ability to answer all their questions, they denied my request and said that I could get another 6 hour pass. I was really disappointed and frustrated. I had followed all the rules and did not create any trouble. I simply could not understand why I was being denied this request. It was a religious holiday and I felt as though my religious rights were being denied. Despite this, I said I would take the 6-hour pass and go to church.

    As I was getting my church clothing ready, I decided that I was going to lie to the nurses and tell them I was only going to church and hanging out with people at the church. However, I decided that I was going to return on Sunday after church and deal with the consequences later. However, in order to do that I needed to pack some clothing but I could not bring much with me because it would look suspicious. So, what I did was wear three layers of clothing including my church dress and packed a small backpack with my laptop and all my electronics.

When I was about to the leave the hospital, I was so nervous. I did not want to get caught. Thankfully, I did not get caught and was able to leave without any problems. When I left the hospital, I decided that I would treat myself to a night at the hotel I visited it. I was able to afford it because my ODSP cheque came and was deposited into my account. I paid for my room and went up. The first thing I did was take a shower. It felt so good. I washed my hair and took the longest shower that I could. It was beautiful. I walked around the room in the hotel robe and towel on my head and felt like a queen. I took a photo and was about to post it and then remembered that people would know where I was. I did not want to be located. I just wanted to have a good time in the hotel. Then the word LEAVE went across my mind. LEAVE the hotel and LEAVE the province and escape to Montreal. I thought to myself that this hospital was never going to let me leave and it was time to leave Nova Scotia.

I quickly went onto my computer and looked up the VIA Rail train service. I looked for the next train out of Nova Scotia to Montreal. The next train was coming at 12:00pm and I had an hour to get there. I quickly got dressed and went straight to the VIA Rail. I had a map and decided to walk to save money. I learned from the past how to stay hidden so I turned on airplane mode on all my devices. I would have used the GPS to find the location but I could not risk it. I checked my time and I had not arrived so I decided to get a taxi. The taxi rushed to the VIA and we made it just in time for me to buy my ticket and board my train. I was so nervous and prayed that I would not get caught. I was so tempted to turn on my Wi-Fi but it was so important that I stay hidden. The train arrived and I boarded the train. I was escaping; I was really doing it.

This was my first time on the VIA Rail and I was excited and nervous at the same time. I just wanted to get out of the province of Nova Scotia so that I could be safe. I knew that if I made any calls or went online that I could risk getting caught by the police and sent back to the hospital. As the train passed city-to-city and closer and closer to the New Brunswick boarder, I became more and more excited. Finally, we arrived in New Brunswick. I was so excited because I was safe. The police couldn't touch me; I was out of their jurisdiction.

Immediately, I turned on my phone and made a phone call to the hospital. One of the nurses on duty answered phone and greeted me. I responded, *"I'm calling as a courtesy to let you know that I have escaped from the hospital and I'm not coming back. You won't be able to catch me because I have already left the province. I just thought I would let you all know as a courtesy."* The nurse paused on the phone and said, *"You won't be coming back?"* *"Yes, that's correct. I'm tired of your hospital and needed to leave. Like I said, this was just a courtesy call. Take care."*

I hung up the phone and started to chuckle to myself. She must have been pissing her pants. What were they going to do? I outsmarted them. I was on the winning side.

Since I was out of the province, I turned on the Wi-Fi on my computer and phone and started to post on social media again. I started to talk about my new home, Montreal. I talked about how thankful I was to be out of the hospital and on my way to Montreal.

To me, Montreal was a beautiful place. In Montreal, I had a friend from high school and was looking forward to seeing him when I arrived. Everything was going to be good. I continued to post on social media about everything. I must have posted at least 100-200 photos and videos on Instagram listing my location.

While on there, a young man in the night messaged me online. He thought my posts were pretty cool and wanted to chat. He was from Nova Scotia. We messaged each other back and forth for at least one hour. Then suddenly, he says, *"what did you do? Your face is all over the news!"* I replied, *"I escaped from the mental hospital and I'm on my way to Montreal."* He started to laugh and responded, *"Holy S**t!"* I decided to Google my name and found an article of me by CBC News and the Halifax Chronicle saying that I was a missing patient and I was in danger because I had not taken my medication. The photo they used was a photo that was taken at the mental hospital with me wearing used clothing and my fur hat. I was upset that they chose to use this photo because it made me look crazy. However, I laughed and continued to chat with this young man for another hour and then I went to sleep.

Since I was still in my used clothing and fur hat that I escaped in, I decided to change my clothing. I went into the restroom on the train and changed into my custom made dress with a big floppy black hat. Once I was done, I went back to my seat and by this time it was morning. Within an hour, the train finally arrived into Montreal and I was so excited. As I un-boarded the train, two Montreal police came up to me and called me by name, *"Ms. Crawford, can you please come with us?"* I pointed to my bags and replied, *"Here are my bags, thank you."* I walked up the escalator and waited for the officers to grab my bags. They led me to their police car and put my bags in the trunk. Although it was customary, they didn't put handcuffs on me. They then opened the back door to the squad car and led me in.

I asked them where they were taking me. They told me that they were taking me to the police station and then to the hospital. They continued to say that there was alert out for me. They asked me why I left Nova Scotia. I told them that the hospital sucked and that Montreal was better. They chuckled and continued to drive. Although I was with the police, I was happy to be out of that hospital and in Montreal. We finally arrived in the police station. They led me out and took my bags out of the trunk. I walked into the police station where there were many other officers speaking French. The admission officer asked me many questions, took my photo and then fingerprinted me.

Once done, I was led into a holding cell until the ambulance came. The ambulance took over an hour to arrive. When they finally arrived, the paramedics checked my vitals and then left for the Montreal General Hospital.

I arrived at the Montreal General Hospital and waited with the paramedics for the admitting nurse to see me. After an hour, I went in and the paramedics gave them my vitals and then left. I was told to change my clothing. They gave me a hospital shirt and pants to wear. I tried it on and as usual, the pants did not fit. I told them and they gave me the largest size. I tried it on and it was very tight but it was bearable. They told me that the hospital was backed up and that I wouldn't be able to go into a room but had to wait in the hallway on a stretcher. I was disappointed but waited nonetheless.

I met a few people there and started to talk with various people in the hallway. There was one Jewish woman who was elderly who I grew attached to. She told me about kosher food and that you could request it if you were Jewish. I decided to request it as well because at that time, I believed I was an original Hebrew Israelite. I told the nurses that I required kosher food and they questioned me. I told them that I was both a Christian and a Hebrew Israelite but would like to exercise my rights as a Jew. They finally decided to change my food order into kosher food. They brought our food and we started to eat and chat together. We chatted for hours and we became friends. We even exchanged addresses. I started to call her my Jewish mamma.

The following day it was time to eat and they didn't have any kosher food. My Jewish mamma was very hungry so she called her husband. When her husband came, he ordered a very expensive pizza and shared it with me. It was the best pizza that I had ever eaten. It cost just over $50 and I couldn't believe it.

While in the hospital, I would post on social media about everything including my treatment at the hospital. I spoke about doctors and nurses and the security team. I talked about how they were treating other patients and much more. One post was about a few doctors. I posted all night long for a few nights. One of the posts I made was of my poop telling the doctors that their careers would be flushed down the toilet like my poop. Well, unfortunately, my posts got the attention of the hospital HR department. The nurses and doctors found out that I was posting information about them and came to take my device away. I became ballistic. I told them that they were not taking my iPad. They called the security and said that I was becoming irrational and needed something to calm me down. I did not want to give them my iPad because I was also listening to music on it and it was my therapy. If they took that away from me, I would have no therapy and no way to communicate to the outside world about the treatment I was receiving in the hospital. The security officers grabbed me and pulled the iPad from me and dragged me into the isolation room. They then proceeded to strap me down and gave me a needle. I started to cry as I felt as though my rights were being violated. I stayed in the room for many hours strapped to the bed. I couldn't believe what they were doing to me. Hours later, they asked me if I would comply and I told them I would. They released me from the isolation room.

After a week of being down in the Emergency department, I was sent upstairs to the psychiatric ward. It was a beautiful ward but unfortunately most of the people spoke French and I did not understand them. They told me that I had to put on different scrubs. It was difficult to find scrubs that fit me due to my size. I finally found something. It had been days without my music and I was feeling weak. I started to sing to myself to keep me calm and relaxed. Later that evening they had a time when everyone on the floor would walk back and forth through the ward while pop music would play. When I heard the music, I went wild. I started to dance my way up and down the hallway. People saw my energy and would dance with me. This made the nurses upset. I guess they wanted us just to walk and be tranquil. So, one of the nurses came to me and told me that I had to stop dancing or they would give me something to calm me down. I stopped dancing but I continued to sing.

On this floor they had different activities including something they called Music Therapy and Art Therapy. When I saw them on the schedule, the creative artist in me became excited. I attended the music therapy class and for the first time I was able to put a description to what music was for me. It was my therapy and I did not know that it took on this form. I was truly thankful to that hospital for showing me this. I remember entering the class so excited. They had various hand held instruments that we could play. We would sing various famous songs like songs from John Lennon,

Bob Marley and Queen. It was awesome! I started to sing a solo of **Amazing Grace** and was joined by a young black boy who had an amazing voice. Go figure, two black people that can sing. I also attended art therapy and created a collage of things I loved. It was also a wonderful class.

As much as I did not want to be hospitalized, I was really enjoying my time there. I carried some Bob Marley DVDs with me and would play them in the DVD room and sing to the music. It was awesome. However, eventually, I wanted to go home. It had been two weeks that I was at the hospital and I was ready to leave.

Since I had been there more than 3 days, I was given the opportunity to see an advocate and obtain a lawyer. The hospital wanted to keep me there for another 30 days and I wanted to appeal that decision so I got a lawyer to fight it. We went before the courts and unfortunately, we lost. I was told that I had to spend another 30 days in the hospital.

However, I was given the choice to where I would spend those 30 days. It would either be that I go back to Nova Scotia, I stay at the hospital in Montreal or return back home to Ontario. I chose to go back home to Ontario. I was so thankful. I spoke to my spiritual mother Karen and my friend Donna about this arrangement. In order for them to send me via bus, I had to have someone that would pick me up from the bus terminal and take me directly to the hospital. I arranged for Karen and Donna to pick me up. It was very early in the morning when I arrived. I arrived around 2:30am. They were so happy to see me safe and sound and took me to the hospital. However, when I arrived, they intake nurse said that they did not have to enforce the 30 day stay because it was from a different province. They said that they would assess me and if they thought I was well enough, they would send me back home. Well, after they assessed me, they determined that I was fine and could go home.

The following day, I contacted the hospital in Montreal to tell them that CAMH rejected me and said that I did not need to stay in the hospital. The doctors there were so pissed. They wanted me in the hospital and started to regret that they gave me the option to return to Ontario.

Back in Ontario, I did not have a place to stay, so I went to stay with my father. He was not happy at first but eventually got over it. I stayed at my dad's house for two months and then became ill again for two weeks. My father did not know how to deal with my mania and wanted me in the hospital. I was making all types of posts about the illuminati and the police and my father grew concerned. While there the police had been looking for me because of my posts. I kept saying that I was going to sue the police for the death of my sister and for harassing me. My dad just wanted me to get better but did not know what to do. Finally, my mania came down and I was doing much better. Though my mania came down, I started to fall into a depression. All I would do is sleep. The medication caused me to gain weight, sleep all the time and have these weird dreams. It was messing with me.

Living with my father put me in close proximity to an old friend's mother, Hakima. I went over to visit her to catch up on old times and found out about her side business. She was selling scarves and dresses from Dubai. They were beautiful Islamic wear that were great for indoors and great as hijabs or pashmina scarves. I told her that I believed I could sell her products and she was excited. With this excitement and her trust in me, she decided that she give me about $250 worth of product to sell on consignment. She would give me 50% of the sales. I thought it was a great arrangement as I was looking for ways to get back into fashion as an entrepreneur.

However, one thing about having bipolar, we always get new business ideas when manic. There is a good chance that I was either hypomanic or manic when I accepted the garments. A few days later, when going to church, I decided to wear one of the dresses with a matching scarf over my head. To me, I looked stylish. However, to others I looked bizarre. This is something that happens when manic. My fashion changes drastically. So, I'm at church wearing this housedress with a head wrap and I received a few stares. I didn't care. After the service, I decided that it was my time to hustle. I pulled out one of the tables and put my scarves and dresses on the table to sell. I proudly stood in front of the table with my Islamic housedress on started to shout, *"Scarves for sale, scarves for sale."* There were a few people that looked at the scarves but unfortunately no one bought one. I was a bit disappointed but did not let that stop me.

On June 25, 2015, I decided that I would make an appointment with my mentor Rathika, the former Member of Parliament of Scarborough-Rouge River. I went there in person to make the appointment. While there, I decided to take a few photos of me in front of a photo with her and the leader of the NDP Party. I also decided to make a video of me in her office to show others that I was there. These videos were important to show my journey and where I had been. I especially wanted to show the police that I was connected to someone in power and they should hence stop harassing me. Once I made the appointment, met with her new executive assistant and finished posting my videos, I left. However, as soon as I left I saw ambulances and police cars coming in my direction. I removed my fascinator and put on my scarf to disguise myself. I figured that the police had recognized where I was and were after me.

I started to run and while searching for refuge, I found a church, the Morningstar Christian Fellowship just up the street from Rathika's office. I figured that it was time that I stopped depending on politicians to help me and it was time that I leaned on the church. I walked to the back of the building and rang the doorbell. They answered the door and let me in. I told them that I needed prayer because I believed the police were after me. They got me to sit down and wait for two individuals that would talk with me. I told them my plight. I told them that I believed that I was missionary and marketplace minister. I explained the death of my sister, my social media activity, and how the police kept appearing wherever I was. I was stressed. They brought me to a room and prayed for me. I felt so much better after I received the prayer. When I left the building, the police and ambulance had left and once again I felt safe.

I decided that it was time that I leave Ontario for Montreal, my true home. I was sick of being harassed by the police and wanted a break from everyone. So, I went back to my father's home to pack a suitcase to go to Montreal. Once my bag was packed, I took the bus downtown to the Toronto Bay Street Bus Terminal. While on my way downtown, I turned off my Wi-Fi on my computer, iPad, and cell phone, as I wanted to slip out of Toronto with the knowledge of the police. I arrived at the bus terminal and bought my ticket to Montreal. Though tempted to turn my Wi-Fi on, I resisted as I felt it was time to leave this place undetected. My bus arrived and I boarded the Megabus to Montreal. I was so excited. I was finally going to be out of this horrible city that I believed had treated me so poorly. While on the bus, I was once again tempted to post on social media about going to Montreal but as I learned last time, don't post if you don't want to get caught. So I stayed on the bus and did not post one thing on social media. This was very difficult for me because I was manic and obsessed with social media. Despite this, I resisted. While on the bus, I tried to find a place to stay and decided to call my friend James from Montreal. Though I didn't get him, I left him a voice mail and hoped he would call me back before I arrived but he didn't. Finally, I arrived in Montreal and felt a sense of relief. I was home my true home.

When I arrived in Montreal, it was in the middle of the night and I needed a place to stay. I decided that I was going to use my Hilton Honours membership card to make a reservation to stay in the Hilton Hotel. Did I have money for the Hilton? No. However, somehow I figured that I would stay there. So, I went to the hotel, used their Wi-Fi, and tried to make a reservation. I had hoped that I could pay my bill when I left but unfortunately, they wanted to secure that amount on my card up front. After staying in their hotel for a while, I was finally asked to leave as they recognized that I did not have money.

I left the hotel and went looking for a place to rest, charge my phone and get Wi-Fi. I found a McDonalds that I was able to do all three. While there, I had a really great conversation with Randzel, a McDonald's employee, about what I do as a social media guru. After about 20 minutes of talking and getting a chance to see his Instagram page, I was impressed and decided that I would make him my Director of Ecommerce and Social Media for my new company. Please note that I did not have a company at present but it was all in my head. However, in my mind it was going to be big. I was going to start my talk show, my new fashion line of menswear and my online university where I teach people about social media. It was going to be big and make me millions if not billions. Another thing I did was change my social media name to CN, short for Cleoni Natacha and drop my last name because that name had brought so much pain in my life. I wanted a new start. A new name would do that for me.

Finally, after hours of being in the McDonalds, I decided to leave and look for a place to stay. I decided that I would make a reservation at the Le **Fairmont** Queen Elizabeth, the most expensive hotel in Montreal. I called them and made the reservation for later that day and for July 18th and posted the details on my social media. When I arrived at the hotel, I went to the President's Club line and requested a new membership card. They gave me a new card, the Wi-Fi code and confirmed my reservation. Though I made the reservation, I knew I wasn't going to stay there that night, as I did not have the money or a credit card. In order for me to stay at the hotel, I needed a credit card that was not a visa debit card. So I told them that I would be going to the bank in the morning and would get a new credit card. This was a lie. I just wanted to be able to leave my baggage there for free while I tried to open an account at the Royal Bank, Scotiabank and run a few errands. They took my luggage and gave me a ticket for them to hold it. After posting a few things on social media, I decided to the leave the hotel.

While in Montreal, I had plans to find a location for my new business. I had plans to sell my scarves, dresses and so much more. I even wanted to start an online university called #ThankUUniversity42 which would teach people how to use social media. I had so many ideas and Montreal was going to be my new home. It was going to be the regional office for my businesses. Though the business ideas sounded good, I was manic and nothing was written down. However, I still believed I had a business. I walked around town with a photo of my business card and the Fairmont hotel membership card in my wallet holder. I used this to show to the various businesses that I would visit. My plan was to become a distributor of various products. I wanted to sell hats, scarves, dresses and various other products from local stores such as men's and women's suits, purses, Adidas original products and much more. In order to obtain these products, I would partner with businesses and sell them on consignment. To do this, I needed a location to house the products.

With that said I started to walk to the Royal Bank so I could open an account and withdraw the money from my Toronto account. I waited in line to open an account and then was ushered by the teller to come forward. I explained that I already had an account and wanted to take out the balance. For some reason, they wouldn't let me take out the balance. I was furious. I started to yell and carry on badly. Suddenly I was approached by a security officer and told to leave. Due to my treatment with officers and security in Toronto, I became agitated and started to resist as my arm was grabbed. I yelled that Royal Bank was racist and that I was taking my account out of there and wanted all my money. They dragged me out of the bank and I grew more and more irate. Then, due to the stress, I fainted and had a seizure. The officers became fearful as they thought they had caused it and were probably afraid that I would sue. I heard them say that they were going to call the ambulance. When I heard that, with supernatural strength, I jumped up and ran out of the building. I knew that if the police and ambulance came, I would be hospitalized again and I did not want that. I fled the building and crossed the road and went into the Scotiabank. While there, I made an appointment to open a Scotiabank account and left the building. When I left, I noticed that the police and ambulance were in front of the building. So, I grabbed my scarf and wrapped it around my head like a hijab and speedily walked up the street.

Eventually, I made it to St. Catherine's Street without being caught by the police. As soon as I arrived, my spiritual mother (at the time), Sis Catherine called me. I told her that I was on her street, St. Catherine's Street. She laughed and I explained my plans for the day. She cautioned me but was supportive. Once the call ended, I posted screen shots of our call and made a bizarre post. I proceeded to visit almost 30 shops and collected business cards as I planned on doing business with the businesses I approached. Some of the businesses, I visited were Apple, Adidas Originals, Moores, and The Bay. Once I was done collecting business cards and finding potential vacant spots on St. Catherine Street, I proceeded to go back to La Reine Queen Elizabeth Hotel. While travelling back to the hotel to collect my bags, I post on social media one particular post was targeted to CBC the television studio. I had written that I love CBC Montreal but as for CBC Nova Scotia, I was going to take them to court and sue them for $4,000,000 for defamation of character for the article they wrote about me earlier that year.

Finally I arrived at the hotel and started to use the Wi-Fi in the lobby. I was then approached by the security and asked to leave. I did not understand why. I started to explain that I had my bags in the back and wanted my bags. They retrieved my bags and asked me to leave. Although I left, I was stressed but decided that I would continue to go window-shopping back on St. Catherine Street. I arrived in Club Monaco and while there, I started to think about how I was treated in the hotel and at Royal Bank and became anxious and fainted. I had another anxiety attack. The staff got me water and I regained consciousness. They wanted to call the ambulance but I requested that they didn't, as I did not want to be hospitalized. Though stressed with no place to go, I left the store.

After fainting in Club Monaco, I decided that it was time to find a place to stay. I found a shelter in the city and was admitted there and spent the night. I was so thankful because it was clean and the people were nice. The following morning, I met a roommate from Congo. She was fluent in French and barely spoke much English. We chatted and I showed her some of my scarves and dresses. I decided to give her one of my dresses as a gift and she gave me one of her dresses from Congo. It was brightly coloured and traditional Congolese wear. I decided to make a head wrap and pocket out of the head wrap. I looked fabulous. As per the dress that I gave her, she mentioned that it was too long, so I took out my sewing machine and started to shorten it. She liked it and kept it. Once we were done trying on each other's clothing, we decided to go for a walk. We visited various hotels and stores. While at each hotel, we would take a photo together and would post the photo on my social media account. Eventually, she became tired and we decided to go back to the shelter for lunch. I asked her if she wanted to come with me again and she declined. She had some friends that she wanted to meet up with so I proceeded to go alone. After spending hours touring the city, I finally made it back to the shelter.

The following day, on June 27, 2015, I discovered that the Montreal Jazz festival was taking place. I decided to rip one of my scarves in two to make a matching headband and scarf. I tied it around my head and wore the scarf around my neck and off to the Jazz Festival I went. I had a great time alone at the festival. It was packed. There was a booth where Bell Canada was taking fun photos with different props. I decided to wear a purple wig and hold a guitar and posed for the photo. I thought I looked great but when I look at the photo on Facebook now, I actually looked crazy. After, doing more sightseeing, I eventually went back to the shelter but called in late. I arrived around 11:30 pm. I arrived past curfew and was told that I would have to leave. I became angry and started throw brochures on the floor. I screamed and threw framed photos and certificates on the ground. I broke glass and smashed drawers all over the place. I started to swear and went into my room and started to gather my things. The police arrived and took me to the police station. From there, I was taken to the hospital. Being as late as it was, I didn't see a doctor till the next morning. I spent the night with my luggage at the hospital. The following morning, I met with the doctor and was released because I knew what to say.

Upon release, I contacted a friend and asked if he could meet me. He picked me up at the Fairmont Hotel and we went to a sports bar. We had an amazing time and then I told him I needed a place to stay. He welcomed me there and I slept on his bed while he slept on the floor. He was a true gentleman. The following morning, I took a shower and continued to roam the streets and do some more site seeing. This time, I was searching the city for places that I could rent for my business. I gathered a few numbers and would take photos of various buildings and post them on social media. There was one building with the numbers 666. I stopped there and considered it to be a cursed building due to the numbers. I made a video and posted it and then I heard a police siren coming and assumed that the police were after me again. So I turned off my Wi-Fi and ran down a side street in fear. Right then and there, I decided that I was done with Montreal and wanted to go home. Since I did not have any money, I called a friend from Ontario and asked if they could send me money to go home. She was concerned about me and sent the money. I went back to my friend's house, gathered my things and was given a ride to the bus station and went back to Ontario.

On July 1, 2015 and I decided to post on social media about my experience in Montreal. I wrote as follows:

"I just got back from Montreal and I am so thankful I went. I got so much inspiration, from the people, the fashion, the colours, the hotels, everything. Even though, I was sent back into a mental hospital for the 9th time this year, the trip was still worth it. I see things so much clearly now that the rain is gone. All of the obstacles are out of my way. (#musictherapy42 break) So, on Friday July 17, 2015 at the @gospelcafeca, #CNCleoniNatacha, formerly #CleoniNATACHACrawford will be launching the concept of her new business and hosting a kick-ass #MusicTherapy42 party with a fusion of musical selections handpicked by me. Tickets are $30 including food. This event is no longer a goodbye party but a hello party to the new me, #CNCleoniNATACHA. No heels allowed, dress your best but you must wear flats or runners. This is gonna be an epic party and wi nuh wan nobody fi leave dis yah party because dem foot ah bun dem! Ah woy! #danceparty #music #motown #steviewonder #supremes #disco #70s #60s #80sbabies #babyboomers #zoomers #getYoGrooveOn - #hashtagcity - #ThatIsAll – Cleoni Crawford @iamjob42"

I then tagged everyone from the @huffingtonpost to @barackobama. Though released from the hospital and now back home, I was still manic. That same day, I met with my spiritual mother, Catherine and made a funny video. How she didn't notice my antics was another question. However, as I look back, I realize that I was still operating at a high. I continued to post on social media things that I thought would build followers and promote my new business (which was many over the past few years while manic), @iamjob42 and my new personal Instagram page

@cncleoninatacha. I posted daily collages of things and people that I had met on social media, places I had been or music that I had been listening to. It was constant and non-stop posts. When I would travel on the subway and arrive at particular stations that had special significance like Queen, I would post a photo of myself in front of the words QUEEN to exemplify that I was the next #CaribbeanQueen. In my mind, I was social media royalty and I wanted to the world to know this.

I was so excited about my new business that I felt like I needed an assistant. So I shared my vision with my good friend Dawn. She was my cheerleader and I love her for that. I decided that I would make her my assistant and she agreed. I also told her that she would start her ministry as well with my help. She was excited. To show this new partnership, we did a mini photo-shoot in her basement wearing my hats and scarves. This photo-shoot represented the various items that would be sold as the COMMERCEandMARKETPLACE minister. I was going to be rich and living my best life. However, though I was a minister of commerce, that wasn't my only title, I was a social media minister, engineer, strategist, musical chemist and teacher. In order to become a teacher, I told myself that I was going to leave Canada eventually and apply to school in Jamaica to study music and get my doctorate so I could teach music. Music had meant a lot to me and had been my therapy and I wanted to travel the world as a social media strategist, teacher, and businesswoman. I believed I could do and have it all.

Another thing I discovered while in Montreal was my name. I was determined to change my name to CN-Cleoni NATACHA. I chose the name CN after seeing the Canadian National Railway (CN Railway) in Montreal. I believed it was prophetic. It was named
after me, Cleoni Natacha the prophet and Queen. Also, I had

determined that my last name was a slave name that was yoked with pain and curses and I wanted to wear my new name of royalty, Madam CN. So, what did I do with this revelation, I posted on social media a picture that said, *"Hello, My name is CN-Cleoni Natacha"* and that I would be official changing my name the following month for the purposes of branding.

While living back at my father's home, I would continue to post on social media and one day while posting, I decided to teach my little brother how to use social media. However, my father had been learning about my activity on social media from his friends. Some of my posts were positive and others had me talking about suing the police and other people. Sometimes I praised and other times I would cast curses on people. I remember being in the living room with my brother showing him social media and my father walks in and asked what I was doing. I told him and he blatantly said, *"He is too young for social media!"* From that day on, I realized that my father did not support the things I did on social media. Despite his support, I continued to post on social media but without my family.

The following day, I decided to go to First Friday's hosted by Warren Salmon. First Friday's is a black networking group of professionals and entrepreneurs that meet monthly with different topics. Prior to attending, I contacted Warren and asked if I could get a table to sell my scarves and promote my social media business. He told me the price and I agreed. To prepare for the event, I went to Kinko's to design and print new business cards. Once done, I went downtown to the venue, which was held at the new East United complex. It was a really great event. People were sharing their businesses and the energy was great. I was dressed in an African blouse from Congo with a matching head wrap. I thought I was appropriately dressed. While at the event, they gave us an opportunity to share our businesses. I went up and shared that I was a social media strategist who was also selling scarves from Dubai at the back. I offered to give a 1-hour free session of social media consulting to the winner of the raffle. A gentleman from Jamaica National bank pulled my card and decided to chat with me after the event. I showed him a few things and took his card to schedule a meeting. Another person I met with a Caucasian lady from Investors Group. We chatted about what she did and I decided to give her one of my scarves. She was very appreciative of it and we exchanged cards. Apparently, she knew how to find finances for businesses and I thought it was a divine appointment for me. While there, I also met an acquaintance, Mr. Fresh of Mr. Fresh air fresheners, who was selling his products to clients.

I took many videos of the event and posted them on social media. The event went to so well that people did not want to leave. We eventually moved our discussions to outside of the building. This was when I met Audia, a woman who hosted a financial literacy conference for young students. Being manic, I was talkative and talked about the importance of young people being financially literate and so much more. I took photos and video of our conversations. We decided to take each other's business card and I was invited to speak at her conference in November. At the end of this event, I was given a ride by my acquaintance, Mr. Fresh, and we had a great conversation about entrepreneurship and making millions of dollars. We were going to be rich. Mr. Fresh was doing very well and had already bought a house at his young age. I was super impressed and knew that I would be next.

The following day, I decided to visit my friends at the Gospel Café for one of their events. It was a concert and I danced the night away. The Gospel Café as said by their name was a Christian restaurant that played Christian gospel music while serving Caribbean cuisine. It was a great spot to be as a Christian.

Once again, I started to promote them on my social media page by videoing their restaurant. That night they played songs like **"I love that man"** and **"Real Real Real"**. It was a really great night.

Chapter 11:
Social Media Queen

It was finally time for church on July 5th. Because I lived so far away, I decided to visit Abiezer Pentecostal Church. The service was really good but it was not like home. I missed my church APC so much that I decided to take the bus to Pickering to attend night service. That week also happened to be consecration week. We were going to be in prayer for the whole week. I would take the bus to and from my father's house to the church all week. God was speaking to me but I was still manic. That same week, I was invited to meet with the same Caucasian woman I met from Investors Group at the prestigious Donalda Club. They had a financial seminar there and I felt like a Queen. To become a member at their club, it cost $50,000 per year. This was a truly prestigious club and I felt like that this was the beginning for me. I felt like I was just about to meet my millions because now I was breaking bread with the millionaires. While there, I secretly took many photos and posted them. It was a great feeling to be there. I could feel that things were about to change for me.

When I arrived home that night on July 9th, apparently the police had visited my father's home looking for me. He was pissed. He did not want any trouble with the law and didn't like what I was doing on social media. I tried to show him but he didn't care. I even explained that I just went to a prestigious club and was about to get my break at really making some money. He didn't care. We ended the argument; I ate dinner and went to bed.

In the middle of the night, I decided that it was time to leave. I was not about to get arrested by Toronto Police. So, I packed my bags and decided that I was going to escape from Toronto and go to Durham. However, before I left, I had to leave my mark in the Humber Summit ward. The City Councillor of that ward had a reputation of being a racist. So, I went to his office and took a photo of me in front of his office for Instagram. In the caption, I posted that he would be cursed and would lose his job because his officer refused to see me. I took many other photos in the dark and cursed the city. I even cursed the construction company that had been working on my grandmother's street because I saw the triangle in their logo, which I determined, was a sign from the illuminati. I left my father's home at approximately 4am. Once again I was fleeing the city of Toronto.

I arrived in Ajax and went straight to the shelter Herizon House. I lied to them and told them I was fleeing my boyfriend who was trying to kill me. I knew that they wouldn't accept me unless I was in danger as this shelter was for people who were in trouble. Though I was not being domestically abused, I was paranoid and felt like the police were harassing me so I left Toronto. I moved into the shelter and stayed in the room called Jennifer at first and then due to my mental illness was moved into a private room called the Scotiabank room. When I moved into this room, I felt that this was prophetic and that I was going to be a billionaire with the help of this bank. The reason I felt this way was because I had learned earlier that year that Nova Scotia was where many blacks lived. I also learned that Scotiabank was in Jamaica and that my father banked at Scotiabank. Therefore, with my mania, I deduced that Scotiabank was the bank of black people and our inheritance. When I think about it now, it doesn't make sense but it made complete sense to me at the time. I continued to post on social media about my anger towards to the

Toronto Police and CBC Nova Scotia. I wrote that I didn't blame the Toronto Police for killing my sister but that I wanted to be left alone. I mocked them for not being able to catch me as I left the city undetected AGAIN. In reference to CBC Nova Scotia, I wanted blood. They had written an article about me that was not a true sense of my character. They had depicted me as "crazy" and I wanted to sue them for defamation of character. For years when you Googled my name you would find information about my work in fashion and now mental health. Now with this article, it is the first thing people see. With that said, I wanted justice. I wanted to sue them for all their money, bankrupt them, and then buy back CBC Nova Scotia as Cleoni Black Crawford Nova Scotia, hence CBC. I had big plans and many lawsuits and I posted all of this on Instagram and Facebook.

Now that I had threatened CBC and the Toronto Police and more, I had decided that I was going to put that all behind me for now. I wanted to embrace my new home Ajax. Ajax was going to be the home of my new business @iamjob42 The Global Superstore and my new realty and hotels business called #HappyHome42. My plan was to get settled into the shelter and then do my walk about in the city of Ajax. I wanted to find the information on the city councillor, MPP, and MP. I needed to find the banks and a retail space for my new store. I had so many plans for the city. I wanted a fresh start and Ajax was just the place to get it. I decided to take a walk and went all of over Ajax South. I walked and took pictures of me in front of the City Hall, Tim Hortons, the Harwood Plaza, the bank and even empty retail spaces that were potential office spaces for my new business. I ended the day by making another post about celebrating #Shabbat or the Sabbath at a Seventh Day Adventist Church in the morning and ending it in truth at my home church

APC for the conclusion of our consecration services. Around that time I viewed myself as a Black Jew and Christian. I called myself an Israelite and as an Israelite I was supposed to receive an inheritance or reparations in the form of my lawsuits and grants. Living in Ajax was going to bring my inheritance. However, in order to get this inheritance, I needed to be in touch with my Hebrew self and do what a Black Jew should do. One thing I wanted to do was visit a Jewish Synagogue. I found the address of one in Toronto but was very hesitant on going back to Toronto considering that the police were looking for me again.

The following day, I went to the Seventh Day Adventist Church up the street from the shelter. The service was nice but the people weren't. They didn't pay much attention to me as a new visitor. They led me to a seat but after service, they didn't greet me or introduce themselves. However, I decided to introduce myself to the Pastor. I gave him a card and told him that I was a social media strategist. I told him I could help his church with their social media help if they needed. He said he would think about it and then I left the church. Before leaving I took a photo of me in front of the church for my next Instagram and Facebook post. It was a beautiful sunny day, so I decided to continue to walk around the city until it was time for consecration service. I went to APC and the service was really good as they talked about not being condemned. I needed that.

The following day, I went to my church APC for Sunday service. It was a TWB Sunday or a Together We Build campaign Sunday. They mentioned the building fund and how we were not approved by the big five banks and needed God to open a door so we could continue building. To show my support, I decided to post on Instagram an open letter to the big five banks by tagging the post to each bank. I mentioned the church, their books, how investing in them had changed my life and how it would benefit their bank. Then, I took 13 donation slips with the packages to give to 13 special people. You see 13 had a significant number to me. It signified the 13 bloodlines of the Illuminati. I believed I represented the 14th tribe and bloodline that was going to crush the illuminati through my lawsuits. At the end of service, I started to post about politicians. Specifically, I posted about my former MP Judy Sgro and the current premier at the time, Kathleen Wynne. I wrote the following:

"Try every spirit! #Women can be used for #God and/or the #Devil. #Premier #KathleenWHYNNE is being used by #Satan to divide families and #corrupt #children through #education. #MemberOfParliament #YorkWest #JudySGRO is being used by #God to #administer #Justice and #morality in #YorkWest. Pray AGAINST THE REPROBATE PREMIER UNTIL SHE BECOMES WORSE THAN #ROBFORD. She is operating by the #principality #Jezebel. Read her bio in #Revelations2verses18to29."

Another post I made was about my business going worldwide. I said I would make a million dollars and then a billion dollars. I urged the church to stop thinking small and remember that we are joint heirs with God and that God was not poor so we should not be. I was convinced in my new millionaire status and that it was just a matter of time.

Though I believed that I would be a millionaire, I decided that I should postpone the launch of my business at the Gospel Café. With this being cancelled, I decided to cool down on social media for a while and did not post till September. I was discouraged and disappointed that I was not able to follow through with yet another plan that I had tried to execute. I started to become depressed and suicidal. My high was coming down and I would lose enthusiasm for life. I was starting to realize that I was living in a shelter and felt like a failure. I tried to hang myself in the room but there wasn't anything sturdy that I could tie my scarf to. Since that was not an option, I would visit the lake and look at the water and fantasize about jumping in. Though tempted, I did not jump. Things were just getting hard for me. At first, I was thankful to be in Durham and in the shelter but now being there for as long as I had been was becoming a problem for me. I desperately wanted a place of my own. I contacted many apartments in the Durham region and even tried to get housing to no avail. Things looked bleak.

Then one day while visiting a place in Scarborough, a 5-minute walk away from my former basement apartment, I decided to go and visit my former neighbours with my spiritual mother Catherine. While visiting there, we saw a FOR RENT sign and I became excited. I spoke to the landlord Cico and begged him if they would take me back. He said he would talk to his wife about it and get back to me. My spiritual mother tried to convince him that she would provide support to me to help keep me on track and he started to be convinced. I asked if I could show her the place and he said it was okay. When she saw the place she loved it. We prayed over the place and claimed it. We left and went back to Ajax to the shelter. While driving to the shelter, I shared how this was definitely God opening a door for me and giving a second chance. I could not believe that by looking at another place literally 5 minutes away resulted in us discovering a former residence available again for renting. This was by chance but divine. I claimed it and believed by faith that the wife would say yes. I called on Sunday and the wife Beryl after giving her conditions agreed to take me back. She also let me know that her husband was against it but she wanted to give me a chance. I was so grateful and thankful.

I told the shelter that I had found a place and would be moving on September 1st. They were so happy for me that they gave me 4 boxes of stuff for my new apartment since I had lost all of my furniture and utensils. They also arranged for me to get $1600 from the Housing Stabilization Fund to get a new bedroom set and more. I was so thankful for all the help Herizons House gave me to help me get back on my feet. I moved and felt a sense of relief. I was home; I was literally back home.

It had been over a month and a half since I had been on social media. Then, on September 10th, 2015, I decided to post the following:

> *I have been offline for a while as I have been reflecting over my life and the challenges I have been experiencing with my mental health. After being hospitalized 9 times this year in three provinces, I no longer had the strength or desire to keep pushing. I told myself, 'you're just going to be a failure anyway. So just hang yourself and kill yourself,' Sounds drastic? Well that is what failure mixed with depression looks like. This time away has given me a lot of clarity and meaningful relationships.*
>
> *Not all could handle my journey, so they exited. I'm not mad at any of you because mental illness is not always a picnic to be around. Trust me, I know. I have to face myself in the mirror daily. Thankfully, I did not hang myself. Thankfully, I did not jump in the lake in Ajax. Thankfully, I made it. I am here. Once again, I will rise. I thought there was no hope of turning this around but I serve a God who I call Jesus who specialized in cleaning up people mired in a pile*

of poop. I know I have burned many bridges but I know a God who can and will turn my life around. I want to thank my Pastor and church @apcministries for not turning their backs even after some of the horrible things I said while unwell. APC Ministries and Pastor Castor you are a perfect example of what love looks like with legs. I conclude to say, if you have failed many times have a gotten tired of your failures, I want to introduce you to a man that specializes in cleaning people buried in s**t. He is cleaning mine and he can clean yours too. I present to you my best friend, Jesus the miracle worker. See you all in a few weeks as I spend more time in the presence of Jesus while working on rebuilding my talk show #HappyHome42. I have a dream. It has been delayed but NOT DEFERRED. Coming soon in 2016, #HappyHOME42. Shalom."

When I posted it on Facebook, I tagged 68 people and 27 liked the status and 11 people commented positive words. My baby sister Feleisha wrote an encouraging post, which said:

"I wanna take the time to say Cleoni Crawford, my big sister; I love you with all of my heart. In my eyes, you are a soldier! Keep fighting and show the world that you will not let your mental illness take control of your life. People might have given up on you, but I definitely will be the sister I'm supposed to be and never turn my back on you!"

These words were so uplifting because I had felt down on myself for quite some time. With that post, she got 55 likes and 15 comments of support. It truly felt good.

The following day on Friday September 11, 2015 was the beginning of Ladies Conference and I was so excited. We had a guest speaker coming in from UPCI World Network of Prayer in

St. Louis, MO, Minister Flow Shaw. Our ladies president had hyped up the event a lot and I was looking forward to getting some prayer for my mental illness. I just wanted to be delivered completely of my illness. So I went to the evening service and it was so phenomenal. Minister Shaw spoke on the subject *"Top Hat"*. As usual the sermon was streamed live on livestream and it touched me. During the sermon, I took a photo of her at the platform preaching, edited it in the pic stitch app by adding different captions such as the date, the scripture verse, the words #HappySHABBAT, @apcministries, the title and the words in honour of 9-11, *"14th Anniversary of 9-11, We Remember."* Once the service was done, I thanked her for the sermon and showed her a photo of it. She gave me the thumbs up and I posted it online on Instagram and Facebook. Once again, I felt like my old self again, doing what I loved which was posting on social media the good things rather than my rants.

The following day, being so excited for Day Two of the sermon, which was an early morning session and lunch with just the women, I prepared a gift for the visiting minister to show my thanks. I could not wait another minute to get to church, as I really wanted to show my gratitude to Minister Flo. I got ready and left my Scarborough home for Pickering by bus. It usually took just over an hour to get there but I did not mind. I remember calling my spiritual mother and for some reason, we got into an argument and my heart rate started to increase. This had been happening a lot to me and I did not understand what it was at the time. However, I think it was the start to my anxiety attacks. I remember yelling with her and then hanging up the phone. I called the ambulance crying and explaining my symptoms. They asked where I was and I told them that I was walking to church. They then said they would meet me at the church. I met them at the church in the parking lot and they checked me out and I was feeling better so they left. Though fine, I was still upset but calm until I saw my spiritual mother enter the building. I was speaking to another sister about what happened and then pointed at my spiritual mother and said, *"I'm feeling this way because of you."* She pulled me aside and basically told me that she was not going to have me act up and embarrass her, as she did not like confrontation. She was a quiet woman and I realize that I was overreacting at the time now but then, I felt it was all her fault. Suddenly, I started to yell in the hallway about women not being able to fellowship and women being haters and then fainted. The sisters surrounded me, got me back to consciousness, and sat me up on the sofa in the lobby. I was upset but calmed down. We then went downstairs for breakfast. During breakfast, I went over to Sis Flo and told her how much I appreciated her that I wanted her to have this gift. It was a book, a scarf from Dubai, and a head covering. I was so excited to give this to her. After breakfast, we went into service for the morning session. It was a really great seminar and I forgot about the whole situation with my spiritual mother. I left church and went home.

    While at home, I do not remember the complete details but I remember feeling very upset about what had happened at church and that I needed to fight my illness. I was sick and tired of its grip on my life. Also, I remember seeing something the night before in the altar that rubbed me wrong. I called it strange fire and made a Facebook post about it. I was sick of sin and it being in my church and churches worldwide. Not realizing that I was becoming manic again, I decided that I was going to wear pants (which are not normal for me), my new hiking shoes, my Jeans Marines pullover jacket, and my Jamaican Rasta hat and dark sunglasses. I had received a revelation about a particular church brother was smoking weed in the church and it crossed my spirit. So, I took a big piece of white paper and rolled it into a giant spliff (marijuana cigarette). I stuffed it with cotton and coloured the edges with a pink highlighter to signify the fire on a joint. I did this because I was going to mock those weed smokers in the church and declare war on its sinful grip on their lives. I wanted blood. Also, I was so hot and angry in the spirit about my mental health that I said within myself that I was going to take my medication and pour it on the altar to signify that I was healed and that Satan did not have any hold of me. I was angry and I wanted to engage in spiritual warfare. I was going to church but not as a pretty saint but as a warrior and judge. Like Rizpah in the Bible, I was about to get all gangster in the spirit and wanted my physical to match it. I remember blasting up my gospel rap music that talked about sin in the camp. I was hyped up and ready to fight so I left my home for battle.

    I arrived at church pretty late in service and walked through the front doors with my dark glasses on and my make-believe spliff in my mouth down the middle aisle straight to the altar. I took out the paper spliff out of my mouth and placed it on the altar and opened the cap of my medication bottle and began to pour the remaining pills on the altar. As soon as I was done, a church brother that I had many confrontations with approached me and I was ready to fight. I turned to him and told him not to touch me or I would punch him. He was trying to calm me down but all I remember is both of us on the floor and the whole church gathered around started to pray and yell in the spirit. They were trying to cast out the devil out of me because I had become violent. They tried to pray for me and I was defiant and started to swear and curse while on the ground. The ladies president came to me and tried to calm me down and I spit in her face. The men tried to stop me because I was fighting but they couldn't stop me. Somehow, they got me up off the ground and then, it happened, I had a panic attack and started to have a pseudo-seizure on the altar due to all the stress. The church continued to roar in prayer and shouting out the devil out of our midst.

I regained consciousness and was led out of the altar to the back of the church where I met my spiritual father Minister McHugh since my Pastor was not in town. Minister McHugh tried to calm me down and he succeeded. He was a man that I had a great deal of respect for so I listened to him and calmed down. I left the sanctuary into the hallway and my spiritual father started to talk to me calmly and get me to relax and then the ambulance and the police came. The ambulance checked me out and I was doing better. Minister McHugh asked me what I wanted to do and I told him I wanted to go back into service but that I would behave.

He was considering it when suddenly the police officer approached me and said he wanted to talk to me. Both Minister McHugh and I were shocked that the police was called. He thought the situation could have been handled without them. However, the officer continued and said, *"Ma'am the people here do not want you here."* I told him to get the *"f**k out of my church."* He continued, *"Ma'am you need to leave."* I told him to get the f**k out of my face and warned him to leave me alone. He continued to jeer me on and then I spat in his face. In anger, he grabbed me and tackled me to the ground and handcuffed me. *"That's it b***h, you're under arrest."* It was raining and the officer began to lead me outdoors as my spiritual father stood by helpless and said, *"Is this necessary?"* I was resisting arrest the whole way to the cop car. When I arrived at the cop car the officer tried to put me in the car with no success, so he slammed me on the concrete payment with my face to the ground in the rain while I sobbed. I was both angry and upset. The two officers together picked me up off the ground and threw me into the car. While in the car, I started to swear at the officer and make threats at him and his children. I started to taunt him and tell him that I'm going to get my people to find him, torture him, and pistol-whip him. Then, I told him that I was like the mafia and that I would have one of my guys come over to his house and shoot his wife in the p***y and torture her. Then, at the end of torturing them, I was going to burn down his house and cause him to lose his pension and become broke. I said so much stuff that the officer got so upset and said, *"Shut the f**k up b***h."* I think he was angry and scared because he actually believed that I would do everything that I said.

We arrived at the station and I was put into a holding cell. I started to reflect on the night. My arm started to hurt. When the officer grabbed my arm, I felt like it was sprained. I wasn't sure so I yelled, *"I need to go to the hospital. The damn officer broke my arm."* I then asked to speak to a lawyer. They granted me that right. The lawyer asked me a few questions about what happened and then told me that the church was not placing any charges, so they most likely will send you home with a warning. Eventually, after being in the cell for two hours, another officer came into give me my conditions of release. One of the conditions was that I not return to my church without permission and the other was that I stayed away from the officer and his family due to the type of threats I made against his family. Once they let me know my conditions they called the ambulance to come and check out my arm. The ambulance came and put my arm in a sling and off to the hospital we went.

We arrived at the hospital and it wasn't a long wait to get into a room but it was a long wait to see a doctor. They gave me an X-ray of my arm to see if it was broken. After two hours of waiting, the doctor finally arrived. He told me that there was nothing wrong with my arm and that it was possibly swelling. He then said that they were going to be keeping me at the hospital to be assessed. I knew what that meant. They wanted to assess me for mental health reasons. I told them I did not need their help and started to put on my clothing. The doctor questioned where I was going and called the security. I told him that I was leaving because you racist doctors are always trying to hold me down. The started to walk down the hallway and then came security. They stopped me, grabbed me, strapped me on a bed and gave me a sedative needle to calm me down. The following morning I was transferred from the Ajax hospital to the Rouge Valley Centenary Hospital. This would be my 10th time in the hospital for that year. To say that I was frustrated was to say the least.

I do not remember the details of being in the hospital but I do remember leaving the hospital eventually. The doctors kept me in the hospital for the standard 3 days or 72 hours. I knew the drill. I had no intention on fighting the doctors in the hospital. I just wanted to get out of the hospital and get back to my life. So, I told the doctors what they wanted to hear and got released on Wednesday September 16, 2015. The first thing I did was go back to Pickering and go to the mall. I made a post collage of me, my pastor, the Declare Jesus album cover, the Stop the Funeral album cover from the Gospel rapper The Ambassador and a smiling photo of me showing my medical information bracelet. I was so happy to be out. However, I did not know if I would be allowed to return to church. So, I called the church and left a message for the Pastor letting him know that I was released from the hospital and questioned if I had permission to return to the church. When all of this went down, my Pastor was not aware and was very angry at how the night went. He was very disappointed that the police had to be called and decided that he was going to change how the ushers were trained going forward. He was angry at the church and how they handled me that night. My Pastor finally called me back and told me that as long as I do not create any trouble that I was welcome to attend the church anytime I wanted. He also let me know that despite my illness that I was loved and appreciated. How my Pastor could have been so chill and cool about me returning was so heartwarming.

I returned back to the church on the 18th for Youth service. I was so thankful to be back and not have to worry about being kicked out by the police. I was a bit nervous considering everything that went down but everyone was so loving and kind. They recognized that what had happened at the church was outside of my control. The following day was the church's 2nd annual walkathon and I was back to my normal joyful self. I arrived at church and started to Vlog my experience to show my view of what had happened that day. It was a really great walk to the church's new property, approximately 6.6 km which was a little over an hour walking. I had great conversations with the saints and we took many photos. With the photos I made three collages, took about 53 photos and made a YouTube video chronicling the event that people appreciated.

Things started to get back to normal but I still wanted to be healed of this sickness. So, one day, I made a long post on social media requesting prayer for my mental illness. Over 50 people liked my request and many replied. What I did with this was create a large document with the names of all the people who agreed to pray for me including my church and Pastor with double-edged arrows pointing from me to them vice versa. It was very creative and people liked it. So I made the following post:

"VIRTUAL THANK YOU: I want to give a special thank you to all the people who liked my prayer request and agreed to join me in prayer for my deliverance and healing. I also want to thank the people who joined with me via text message and my church family who joined with me physically. The 21-day fast held at my church has ended as of Monday. Therefore, by FAITH, I believe I am delivered and healed. God has already shown me that he has begun the process as for the first time; I did not fall into a depression after my last MANIC episode. BLESS GOD, that's progress! On a segue, I am very thankful that my Ladies Ministry President, Catherine Heath, was able to see in the spirit on my last manic episode that there was a HOST of demons that were following me. This is CONFIRMATION that my battle with mental illness was not JUST physical but SPIRITUAL. This GREATLY helped in focusing our prayers against both the spiritual and physical elements of mental illness. Furthermore, this also shows me that the mental health field not only needs a DSM book to categorize mental illness but the SPIRIT OF DISCERNMENT. This will prove helpful as God leads me into the mental health ministry. I have faith that the effectual and fervent prayer of you all has played an important role in my healing and deliverance (James 5:16).

With that said, I made this collage which I will be framing in my home, posting in my prayer book as reminders of people I should intercede for regularly, and pasting to my scrapbook to remind me of all the people that joined me in prayer.

I hope from this diagram you will see that prayer is NOT just a one-way thing but two ways. Hence, I pray for you, you pray for me and in the end we sharpen one another (Proverbs 27:17 and Job 42:10). You will never know how much I love and appreciate you all. Thank you for your role in my healing. Love you all."

After I made this post, a few days later, I felt as though I received my deliverance. However, only time would tell if this were true.

Chapter 12:
Kick Push

It had been a few months since my last manic episode and I was thankful. I had just gotten into the RISE program at University of Toronto for people with mental health issues and I was so excited. I really enjoy being in school because it improved my overall mood and sense of worth. I was learning how to write a business plan and would receive mentoring to kick-start my business. I started to post on social media a lot again. However, it was very positive as I was posting about my new business. I wanted to create a new clothing line that would include men's bespoke suits and hoodies and such. I connected with Movember and wanted to design a few hoodies with the mustache on them and sell them in support of men's mental health. However, in regards to the bespoke men's suits, it was only an idea because I did not have the skill to produce such suits. Though I did not have the skill to make it, I planned on finding a tailor that I could partner with. I would sell some suits as bespoke and others I would get from stores like Tip Top Tailors, Harry Rosen and Moores. It seemed like a great idea but I did not think it through yet or finish putting it in my business plan. You see, with my mental illness, I always have ideas for new businesses but I don't always think about the logistics before I start talking about what I'm doing.

Despite this, I continued to post online about this clothing line and the potential launch that would be in February at the Holiday Inn right for my birthday. It would be a dinner and tickets would be $88. I chose the number 88, as I believed that 8 meant rebirths and I wanted rebirth times two. That month, in my hypomanic state, I went downtown very early in the morning to print business cards. It also happened to be Nuit Blanche. So while downtown, I entered a Burger King to the use the restroom and while there met a young man named Jepaul with his friends. We started chatting and I found out that he was a model, so I asked if he would model for me. He agreed and we exchanged Instagram handles and numbers.

My church was just about to celebrate their 20th anniversary and decided to make a beautiful logo. When I saw the logo, I came up with the idea to make a t-shirt for them since I was a fashion designer with their new logo on it. So, I made a digital copy of the t-shirt and posted it on Facebook and Instagram I wanted to sell these shirts as a thank you for helping me to raise almost $1500 towards my talk show #HappyHome42. These shirts would be sold for $20 and all proceeds would be donated towards the Together We Build building fund. I tagged many people from the church in the post and waited for the orders to start rolling in. Since they never rolled in, I decided to go to a t-shirt print shop to get a sample made so I can show everyone that I was serious and that shirts could be made. So, I made the shirt and showed it to my Pastor and Brother Sam and they loved it. However, when it came for the time to sell the shirt, it did not go as planned. Despite this, I did not give up on it.

As I mentioned above, I had another project going for Movember. I wanted to raise money by making t-shirts and hoodies with the mustache on them. I got the shirts and hoodies designs and they were pretty cool. I printed 2 hoodies and 3 t-shirts in different colours as samples to show and get orders. Each hoodie and t-shirt would have your name printed on the back with the number 01 on the back. I was really proud of them. So I showed them to my rapper and church brother Timothy. He really liked them and agreed to help me sell them. We decided to set up a table at church to show these shirts and the APC shirts. Though people liked them, no one purchased. I was disappointed but I kept pushing forward.

I continued to post on social media about different places, hotels and stores that I had visited on social media. I had believed by posting photos of myself in front of these retail stores, banks and hotels that one day that would build my social currency which would in turn make stores want to either sponsor or partner with me. So I would continue to post from everywhere I would visit. While doing I discovered another song that spoke to me. It was Lupe Fiasco's **Kick Push** song. I heard it on BET one day and I fell in love with it. I found the song and downloaded it and played it constantly until I was able to 'freestyle' over it. So, one day, I made a video of me freestyling over my newfound song and posted it because I had believed that Lupe Fiasco was a prophet just like myself. Though I thought it was good, it was just okay but it was just an example of how creative I can become when manic or in hypomania.

A few weeks had passed and it was the end of October so I decided that it was time to promote these shirts more hard by doing a photo-shoot. However, my photo-shoot was pretty ghetto because I did it with my iPhone. So, I called the model that I met in Burger King and Timothy and met at Eaton's Centre. We met in the mall and went to Tip Top Tailors to try on a few men's suits. I also carried my new MY MO moustache hoodies with me. I got Timothy to hold up both hoodies as I took a photo. Then, as both Timothy and Jepaul tried on suits, I would take photos of them for our impromptu photo-shoot. Once we left Tip Top Tailors, we ended the photo-shoot and I posted the photos online. I was so excited about my new clothing line and felt like it was going to sell because of my charitable aspect to it: 25% of all sales would be donated to the organization Movember to promote Men's mental health. I really wanted to support that organization.

Social media was not just an outlet for me to promote my brand and business but an outlet to express my displeasures and happiness about various issues. It was my social playground where I got to meet people I would never meet in real life. It gave me a voice that I had lost due to my mental illness. However, sometimes, that voice was used inappropriately. Around the beginning of November, the Christian organization, the Voice of the Nations wanted to continue to host their annual concert at Yonge-Dundas Square in downtown Toronto and for the first time were denied because they were seen to be proselytizing. There was an outrage about this and I as a Christian was also outraged.

To show my outrage, I looked up the information on the people who were in charge of permitting out Yonge-Dundas and found out that Virgin Mobile Canada was responsible. So, I decided to post on Instagram and Facebook that Torontonians should boycott Toronto and shop in Durham because if the City of Toronto wasn't going to step in they shouldn't get our money. I was livid and decided that not only was I going to talk about it but I was going to take action. I decided to create a hoodie that said #Boycott #Toronto, Shop #Durham and said I was hosting a protest against this at Queen's Park. I made flyers showing their shirt and went downtown in the middle of the night plastering these sheets all over downtown. I plastered it on retail stores, banks, hotels, and even colleges and universities. I felt like I was on a mission and was doing God's work as a prophetess. I was warning the city of Toronto of the judgment and wrath of God that they would experience if they did not permit Voice of the Nations the chance to perform. Though noble, as expressed earlier, it was not my fight. However, in the end the city of Toronto granted Voice of the Nations the chance to host their event. I felt really good about that and made sure that I attended the event the following year.

Though I was using my social media account for good, I started to post excessively. I started to post so much that the media team in my church blocked me. I was super upset about that and did not understand why. However, as I look back, it makes sense why. To me, the posts made complete sense but to others, it looked like I was mad and not making much sense. In one post I would complement someone or posting funny jokes, in another, I could be blasting someone about their sins. My posts were erratic.

With all the social media activity, I was starting to lose sleep. I wasn't getting a full night's rest. I was so focused on getting my business up and running that I was becoming obsessed and driven. Though there is nothing wrong with being driven, the problem is when you don't what is driving you. For me, my bipolar was driving me. I was becoming irritable and defensive and eccentric.

For example, one night while on my way home, I felt that I was on a mission to rid the city of Toronto of the drugs in the city. I was walking down Queen Street at Jarvis where there was a big church. I walked towards the church and discovered that people were smoking crack on the building. Since, I felt I was the city's prophetess. I was sent by God to judge and bless the city and this time it was all about judgement. In anger, I yelled, *"in the name of Jesus, drop that crack! This is God's house!"* Then, I took out my music and started to do interpretative dance and hip hop dancing on the top steps of the church. People were watching me but I didn't care. I believed that I was praise dancing and that by doing this, I would drive out of the demonic spirits out of the city. Strangely enough, as I danced, a woman who was on crack, started to scream out and tell me to leave. I screamed back at her and told her to leave because the Queen of Queen Street was here. Suddenly, a Caucasian man his 40s, approached me, watched in amazement, and asks me why I was dancing. I told him that I was expressing myself. He told me that it was beautiful and he felt drawn to come to the park that night. We started to talk and then a homeless man came and asked if we had any money. I told him no but the other man pulled out $20 and gave it to him. I thought that was kind of him but also foolish considering the neighbourhood and that the homeless man was going to use it for drugs.

The man who approached me then asked if I wanted to get something to eat. I said yes because I did not have any money. We talked and walked and then finally found a place to eat. We chatted about everything and then I told him I needed to go home. The man, whose name was Robert, told me that I seemed like a really nice lady, but I looked tired and needed to get some rest. He was concerned for me. Robert grabbed a taxicab for me and took the cab with me all the way to Scarborough. He told me that I should sleep and he would wake me. Eventually I arrived home; he walked me to my door, wished me good night and went back into the taxi.

I was infatuated with this stranger. No man had ever been soon kind to me. I felt blessed. Though thankful, when I reflect on that night, things could have ended a lot differently. Sadly, with my mental illness when manic, I am very trusting to everyone. Though I shouldn't have been so trusting towards this stranger, I felt like God was protecting me from myself. He knew I hadn't slept in days and that I simply needed to go home.

By now I was 34 and still single. Meeting Robert made me feel like I had potentially met my future husband. I had never met a man like him. He was a photographer and editorial writer. As a woman who loved the camera, he had told me that he could be my photographer. With his card still in my hand, I decided to check him out and found out that he was exactly as he said he was. He was a professional and he made black women look beautiful. I was in awe and decided to write about my experience online. I was feeling gushy inside. It had been a long time since a man made me feel like this. Filled with passion, I got on my social media and started to make numerous posts tagging him and many others. I was obsessed. The following day, I believe that he had blocked me and that was the end of my night and shining armour.

    Though disappointed and still single, I decided to continue my focus on my new business. I contacted Jepaul for another photo-shoot. This time we met Eaton's Centre. When I arrived, I met him and his girlfriend Danica and I told her that we were going to try on a few more suits and clothing from the Adidas store. They were down with it. First, we went to the Hudson's Bay and tried on a few suits. We took photos and posted them on Instagram and Facebook. His girlfriend really loved how he looked in the suits. She went over to him and gave him a kiss and I being the camera happy person I was I took a photo of the moment. I then asked if she wanted to model for me as well as I had t-shirts and sweaters that I needed photos for. She agreed and I got both of them to try on my new My MO clothing line. We took photos of them as a couple in my clothing. Once we were done at The Bay. We went to the Adidas originals store at Yonge-Dundas Square. We took out many items from Adidas and tried them on. I told the staff that I was going to be meeting with Adidas and wanted my models to try on a few stuff for that meeting. They agreed and we continued to try on a ton load of clothing. While there, I also tried on clothing and got them to take photos of me in their clothing.

    Though nice, the Adidas clothing I tried on was pretty tight. I am a full figured woman and Adidas is for slim individuals. Once done, I thanked Jepaul and Danica and let them leave wearing my sample MY MO sweater and t-shirt asking them to promote the brand. I was not thinking at the time because I was manic.

Online, I made it seem as though I was working with Adidas as I created a new logo that featured the Adidas originals logo all around my logo. I really believed that we had a really great business so I posted that we were doing a meet and greet with my new team of models: Timothy, Jepaul and Danica at my favourite restaurant The Gospel Café. I scheduled to have this meeting on Thursday November 12th, 2015. The plan for that evening was to give people a chance to meet us and invest in my business. I was giving people a chance to own 0.5% of #HappyHome42TV. By faith, we were going to be a Fortune 500 company. I was optimistic and was thinking big. However, as days passed, I had to cancel the meet and greet as Jepaul and Danica were no longer interested in working with me. So it was back to square one.

I was tired of people being unreliable and decided that I would feature myself as a brand and spokesperson for my clothing line. I would take photos of myself in the Adidas and C-virtue clothing. I wanted professional photos for my portfolio to show Adidas and decided that it was time to do a professional photo-shoot. After seeing the work of Sean of Sean Anthony photos, I scheduled an appointment with him. Knowing that he was gifted, I was really excited about this shoot. When I arrived to his apartment which he converted part of it into his studio, my excitement grew as time passed. With fast pumping music blaring in the speakers, I started to pose for the camera. We had a lot of fun doing the shoot as I did various poses. I changed three times and showed different looks. It was such as great experience. He gave me the photos that same day, as I really wanted them as soon as possible. After the photo-shoot,

I decided that I wanted to be a plus size model for Adidas. When I meet with Adidas again, I will show them my photos featuring their products.

Chapter 13:
Promiscuous Girl

Once again, I was sent to the mental hospital for my condition and then released because I knew what to say. My medication continued to mess with my system and I desperately wanted a change. So, I went to see my psychiatrist and told him about my condition. He recommended a new drug called Latuda and this was much better but still not good. I took Latuda for a while and it worked for a while. However, although the drug was not supposed to cause me to gain weight, I gained weight. With this medication, I had to take it at night with a meal that had at least 350 calories. With my schedule I found it difficult to take my medication with food and eventually went back to my psychiatrist and requested a new drug. The drug that was recommended to me was Abilify. This drug had little side effects and I was happy with it.

The RISE program was trying to help me turn my idea of a talk show into a sustainable business. After much thought, I decided that I would sell mental health clothing with the Adidas logo on it. In addition, I would sell #HappyHome42 swag like cups, mugs, bags and such. Also, I would host two mental health events annually to bring in income. With these ideas, I found myself at the print shop a lot. I was up all hours of the night working on my business plan trying to get it just right. Finally, after printing a few samples of my shirts and hoodies and having my business plan completed, I was ready to return to the Adidas head office to pitch my idea.

Filled with excitement, I started to post about my potential collaboration with Adidas and that I was going to pitch my idea.
In fact, I started to post only about Adidas. It was obsessive. I guess I wanted Adidas to know that I really believed in their products and wanted to collaborate with a mental health line.

As I would post, I would notice that there were more police cars around me than normal. Despite this, I would continue to post. Then, I would start posting at a spot, turn my Wi-Fi off and leave and watch what would happen. Suddenly, I noticed that police would arrive at the location that I had just left. This is when I started to feel as though I was being followed. I knew that the police had gained insight into where I was in the past by my social media posts and my phone and I truly believed they were trying to harass me again. Realizing how important this meeting was, I decided to turn off my data and Wi-Fi and continued to the Adidas head office. I got off the bus and started to walk when my phone rang. I spoke to the person on the phone and then hung up.

As I continued to walk, I decided that I would stop at the Holiday Inn at the corner of Hwy 27 and Hwy 7. You see I had been visiting various hotels to find a location to host my Adidas themed party. I had visited the Trump hotel and the Fairmont Royal York earlier that week to see if they could be potential spots for my party. However, as I drew closer to the Adidas group, I thought that it would make more sense to have my event closer to the Adidas head office since my party had the Adidas theme. I met with the sales rep for the Holiday Inn and viewed the banquet hall. I loved it. I made a video post showing the room and me talking about potentially hosting my kick ass party there. I took the package, shook hands and left the building. As I left the building, what did I see? I saw a police car parked right outside the hotel. Now, I knew I was being followed. I immediately turned off my data and Wi-Fi and went into airplane mode. To make myself not obvious, I waved at the officers and with my heart beating quickly, walked past their car.

A few blocks up, I saw another banquet hall. I thought I would check it out. When I saw it, I was amazed. They had flashing lights, beautiful fixtures and a large screen. I decided I wanted more information about this location. I met with the manager and told them about my plans to have a big Adidas themed party and wanted to know how much this location would cost. He prepared a package for me, showed me the room again and I took a video and posted it. When I left the building, I saw another police car. When I saw the car, all I could do was laugh. First, the Toronto police were harassing me and now the York Regional police? What the hell was going on? This time, since I was so close to getting to my destination, I turned off phone and started to pray as I walked. If the police were really after me, I was not going to allow them to prevent me from reaching my goal of dropping off my package to the Adidas Group.

Finally, I arrived at the Adidas Group and the first thing I saw was a large photo of Pharrell Williams wearing the iconic Adidas track suit and shoes that he had designed. Considering how much I loved Pharrell and that I thought he was a prophet at one time, I thought that this was a sign that I was destined to be there. I entered the elevator and went to the reception. Upon arrival, I requested if I could see someone from Marketing. The receptionist told me that they do not see anyone without an appointment. I told her my idea and she told me that I could email them the package and wait for them to get back to me. I took the business card and was so happy. I was one step closer to my goal. Though I was done with Adidas, with all the police harassing me, I decided that I needed to leave the city for a break.

With the RISE program coming to an end, I decided that I was going to go to Ottawa and then Montreal and then Jamaica. People were very critical of my social media activity and I viewed them as haters. I was growing sick of Canada. I felt like I was being treated unfairly and harassed by police so I decided it was time to leave again. However, this time I was going to leave to get justice for me. Before that I was going to go to the Adidas head office in Montreal to pitch my business and collaboration with them.

Frustrated with Canada, I bought a ticket to leave for Jamaica on December 27, 2015. Finally, I was going to get out of this country for my true country. Days later, I hopped on a bus destined for Kingston, Ontario. When I arrived I thought it was God showing me a new safe place to stay. You see, I had been thinking of going to Kingston, Jamaica. I thought that by landing in Kingston, Ontario that it meant that my next stop was Jamaica. I believed that it was prophesying to me. First, I travelled along Kingston Road and now Kingston, Ontario. The next stop had to be Kingston, Jamaica, West Indies.

While in Kingston I decided to walk around the city and claim the city by walking by foot. It was extremely cold in Kingston and I wasn't dressed warm enough for this type of cold. However, I continued to walk until I found a Tim Horton's. With frost bitten hands, I entered the Tim Horton's to warm up. With just a few dollars in my account, I bought myself a hot chocolate and donut. I was very hungry. Once warmed up, I left the Tim Horton's and continued walking. Eventually, I found a Comfort Inn hotel and decided that I would go in as I was freezing and needed a place to stay. Though I did not have money for the hotel, I acted like I did. They took the reservation and I said I would be staying for a week. I knew if I had told them that I was staying for the night I would have to pay the whole bill at that moment. However, if I was staying a week, they would only need to secure my credit card for the reservation. So, they took my card and the machine wouldn't work. Considering this, they gave me the key to my room and said we would retry it in the morning. Before leaving, I asked the attendant what time breakfast started. She told me it started at 6am and that it was free and continental. I was elated to hear this, as I was very hungry. I grabbed a cup of hot chocolate and a few free apples and went to my room. When I arrived in my room, I took out my computer and looked up the instructions to find the nearest bus station. I found it and decided that I was going to leave the hotel after breakfast without paying. Once breakfast started, I ate everything they had and took extras for my trip to Ottawa. I changed my clothes into warmer clothing by wearing layers and repacked my suitcase. Casually, I waved to the attendant and I told her I would see her in a few hours. However, I had no intention of returning or paying. As far as I was concerned, I was telling Canada to f**k off.

As I left the building, I saw a bus approaching but I did not have any money. I boarded the bus and told them I needed to get to the bus station but I did not have any money because I was lost. Considering it was very early in the morning and she felt sorry for me, she let me on. She told me that she didn't go directly to the bus station and that I would have to walk 30 minutes to get there from her last stop but she would try and get me as close to my stop as possible. The bus driver continued to drive and drive for about an hour. One by one, passengers would leave the bus until only the bus driver and I were on the bus. Finally, I arrived at the last stop and driver reminded me of how to walk to the bus station. I put my headphones on and started to walk to the station. Thirty minutes later, I arrived at the station. Though tired from dragging my luggage, I was so grateful to arrive.

I entered the Via Rail station and gave a sigh of relief. I searched for an outlet to charge my phone and waited for the train. Though I did not have any money, I told myself that I would board the train no matter what as I was determined to get to Ottawa and then Montreal. I needed to speak to my friend Judy Sgro in government about the harassment I had been receiving in Toronto. I needed justice. Eventually, the train arrived and I boarded the Via Rail and was feeling really good until the ticket collector came. He asked for my card and I gave it to him. It declined. I told him to try it again as I knew I had the money. We tried it again and it declined again. I asked him if he could give me a few moments so I could get in touch with my friends or family to get them to wire me some money. Reluctantly, he agreed. I called my family and friends and one by one they told me that they didn't have money and that I needed to come home. I told them that I was so close to arriving to Montreal and meeting the people at the Adidas head office. Since I was not able to see anyone at the Adidas office in Toronto, I figured I would go to the Montreal office and meet someone there. The passenger in the next aisle close to me apparently had been listening to my conversation. She called the ticket collector over and decided that she would pay my bill. The ticket collector came to me and told me that I did not have to worry about my bill as another passenger paid for it. I was so grateful. It must have been a sign that I was on the right path.

    I arrived in Ottawa and it was freezing. I did not know how cold Ottawa could be in the winter. I went to Parliament to see Judy but met her executive assistant Glen as she was out of town. I explained to Glen my ideas and that I had been harassed by police in Toronto and wanted to leave the country. He listened to me but told me that there was nothing their office could do. He recommended that I got a lawyer instead. He took me downstairs and bought me lunch and set me on my way to go.

I went to the Via Rail station again to go to Montreal. While there I met a gentleman that was very talkative. We started to talk and laugh and he was good company. He had a bottle of wine with him and he offered me some. I declined and told him that I did not drink. He complimented me on my hat and clothing, as I was looking quite posh. His train arrived, he said goodbye and then left. I continued to walk around the station and met this fashionably dressed woman. We talked about the weather and our trips. I explained to her that I was trying to go to Montreal to start my life over again and meet with the Adidas head office. I told her some of my plans and she was impressed. She thought I was cool. I also told her that I did not have any money to get to Montreal and could not get any help from friends or family. She then said, *"You know, I normally don't do this, but I'm going to help you. I'm going to pay for your ticket."* I could not believe my ears. Thankful, I gave her a hug and expressed my gratitude. She paid for my ticket and handed me the ticket and wished me all the best. I looked up to the sky and said a simple, *"thank you Jesus, you are definitely looking out for me."*

The train arrived in Montreal and I was so excited. I was going to leave Toronto and make Montreal my second home; my first home would be Jamaica. Upon arrival, I decided that I needed to find a place to stay. I researched a few shelters and found one. It was outside of Montreal. I was told that I needed to arrive by a certain time that afternoon to secure my spot. I decided to do some site-seeing first and go to the Adidas store on St. Catherine's Street or Rue St. Catherine in French. After a long walk, I finally arrived to the Adidas store. I asked them for the address of the head office and they gave it to me. I was excited because I was getting closer.

I was in the same city as the Adidas head office and this made me feel accomplished. After hours of walking around, I decided to call my friend James to see if he wanted to meet up. I was unable to reach him that day so I went straight to the shelter. I arrived at the shelter and it was this large house in a beautiful neighbourhood. I met with the intake coordinator to discuss why I needed a place to stay. Once I answered all her questions, she accepted me, told me the ground rules and gave me the grand tour. I left my suitcase downstairs and was led to a commons room to wait in till dinner. The room was filled with elderly women and a DJ playing old school music from the 70s, 80s and 90s. I had been under deep stress and music had always been my therapy. Song after song, I started to sing along and then got up and danced to the music. One by one, the elderly ladies would get up and joined me to dance. I grabbed my phone out and started to video myself dancing to the music. They played songs like Whitney Houston, Michael Jackson, Donna Summers, Kool and the Gang and much more. I had a great time with these ladies. Then it was time for dinner. I ate my dinner and was led to see where my room was. I took a shower and went to bed, as I was exhausted.

Although I loved being in Montreal, I had to go back to Toronto to catch my flight. Sadly, I wasn't able to get to the Adidas head office because it was out of town and I didn't know how to get there in time. Thankfully, I receive my ODSP deposited into my account and was able to pay for my ticket back to Toronto. I was so excited to go to Jamaica. I was finally going to escape this horrible cold weather. With my entire luggage in hand, I took the bus to the bus station, bought my ticket and waited for the bus to Toronto. Finally, after 3 hours, my bus arrived.

It was a long bus ride home to Toronto and there was a 3-hour layover in Kingston, Ontario. This station was in the outskirts and

I don't remember if they had any Wi-Fi but I kept myself busy listening to my music, my music therapy.

    I do not remember how it happened but while waiting I had a seizure in the bus station and the ambulance was called. The nearest hospital was in Ottawa so they took me to the hospital in Ottawa. While at the hospital, I waited hours in the room waiting to see the doctor. They told me that I would have to wait a while because it was late in the night and the doctor may not come till morning. Finally, the doctor came and I do not how and why he did this but I was put on a form 1 and transferred to the mental hospital. I was worried because my flight was leaving for Jamaica in just two days. You see I had big plans for Jamaica. With my mania, I had planned to build a 17-bedroom hotel. I would get the money from the Ryerson Start Me Up program, which gave angel investments from $250,000 to $4,000,000 and possibly the Jamaica National bank. Though I did not have a business plan, the idea made perfect sense. Also, I wanted to apply to the University of West Indies and study music. I wanted to spend the latter part of my life as a Jamaican citizen because I was tired of the racism and harassment that I had experience by the police in various cities in Canada.

    While at the hospital, I made many friends or acquaintances and got along with many people because of my singing voice. I loved to sing, as this was how I coped with my difficult situation. Finally, I met with the doctor at the mental hospital and was very anxious. I explained to him that I did not understand why I was being kept in the hospital when all I had was a seizure. He explained that he thought that I was manic and needed to be kept here. I was pissed because by staying I would miss my flight, which was in two days. In my manic state I told him that if I didn't have a flight I would stay but I didn't buy travel insurance and needed to get on that flight.

Furthermore, in anger I asked them if the hospital was going to refund my ticket. Of course, they said no. So I flew into a rage and was once again strapped down until I calmed down. I couldn't believe that I was losing my chance at going to Jamaica.

Unfortunately, I was forced to stay there for six days and missed my flight. While there I met a young man who was looking for a place to stay. His name was Geoffrey. Since I believed that I was going to move to Jamaica eventually, I offered to give him my place to stay. Though I offered him the place, it wasn't my place to offer, as I was only a tenant in the basement. Finally, the six days were up and I was released. Being in Ottawa with all my money spent, I had no way of getting home. Considering this, the hospital gave me a bus ticket back home to Toronto.

Once again I was back in that racist city Toronto and I was not happy. I wanted to be in Jamaica. I had believed that Jamaica was the land of the prophets. To me, the last major prophet in that land was Bob Marley. With my grandiose thinking, I believed that I was the next prophetess and Queen of Jamaica. I was the dancing and singing prophetess coming to bring music therapy to Jamaica. In addition, I was going to use my skills as a social media strategist to work for the Jamaica Defence Force as a social media strategist and decoder. I would finally gain the respect as an officer and a Jamaican. I wanted to deny my Canadian citizenship in exchange for a Jamaican one. However, being in Canada with no money meant that this was no longer a reality.

Depressed by all the opportunities that I had lost, I stayed off of social media for a few weeks until it was close to my birthday. Months before, I had planned to have a big gala for my birthday to launch my business but I decided to cancel it. Instead, I wanted to do something for myself. I wanted to stay at the Fairmont Royal

York for my birthday again. However, this time, I would stay for a week. My plans were to rent up to eight rooms for my friends and I. The only problem was that I did not have the money for that. However, I believed that I would host my music therapy event in June and be able to raise money from that event.

Around that time, the NBA All Star game had come to Toronto. With that said, there were numerous basketball stars in the city. My mania had become out of control again. This time was different; I was highly sexual. I wanted to have sex with everyone. I was sexually aroused all the time. I decided that I was going to go downtown to meet someone to have sex with. I went to a hotel and met a few guys and told them that I was horny. They asked if I would do head which was oral sex and I agreed. He asked me if I would do it on a few people. I thought about it for a minute and agreed. We went upstairs and I went into their hotel room. These men were American and had come for the All Star game. I started to take off my clothes and asked who wanted to get it done. They couldn't believe what they were hearing. Suddenly, one of the roommates came in and said they were no longer interested and I left and went to the bar. I started to chat with a man at the bar. We had a great conversation and I started to flirt with him. He bought me a drink and we chatted. I asked him if he had a room there and he replied yes. I told him that I wanted to have sex and he declined. I asked him why? He replied, *"You're a beautiful lady but I'm gay."* I was so disappointed. Despite this, we exchanged business cards and I told him I would hit him up if I ever went to Chicago as that where he was from. Saddened that I was not going to get any sex, I walked over to the Trump Hotel. I wanted to make a reservation for my birthday. I walked in and tried to make a reservation and was denied from doing so. Then, who do I see, but the one and only Kevin Hart enter the building. I was star struck and wanted to say hello but was stopped by the security. Since I was denied a reservation, I became very stressed by this. Suddenly, I fainted and had a seizure. The ambulance was called and they offered to take me to the hospital. I declined. I just wanted a reservation at the hotel. I was then asked to leave the Trump Hotel. I told them that I would sue them for discrimination and left.

Manic and super sexual, I started to post naked and half naked photos of myself on social media and posted that I was looking for someone to have sex with. Suddenly, I received a response from this cute Spanish guy. He was much younger than me. I had phone sex with him and told him all the naughty things I would do with him. Turned on, he asked me if I wanted to meet him. He picked me up in his Mercedes Benz and we went searching for somewhere to have sex. We went into a building and had sex in the laundry room. I felt so good. It had been a long time since I had sex. Finally I was getting some. I took a photo of him and posted it on social media and called him my Spanish papi. After we were done having sex, he started to get paranoid and thought he was being followed. I told him that it was probably the illuminati, as they like to follow me. This scared the hell out of him. He left me in the building and ran to his car in a panic. He blocked me on social media and that was the end of that.

A few days later, a friend of mine, Mr. Fresh was having a birthday party at this club. It was a great party but I started to feel like I didn't belong so I left. While waiting at the bus stop, an Indian man in a Mercedes Benz stopped at the bus stop and asked me if I wanted a ride. I told him I did because it was almost 2am. He had one condition though. He asked me if I do head. What that meant was he wanted to know if I would perform oral sex on him. I thought about it and being as sexual as I had been, I agreed. Agreeing to this proposition, he zipped down his pants and while driving I performed oral sex on him. This was the first time I had done something like that. Eventually I arrived home and invited him in for some more sex. It was the most boring sex that I had ever had because he was not blessed in that area. Despite this, I pretended that I enjoyed it and then he left.

My sex drive was increasing by the day. I wanted more sex so I would actively seek out men to have sex with. One man I found on the Go train. I flirted with him and told him that I was looking to f**k. He was excited but I told him that I wanted to do it in a hotel since my house was in Scarborough. We searched downtown for a place and everywhere was too expensive. Eventually, we kissed goodnight and I wished him well. The following day, I met this young black guy on the TTC. We started to chat and I told him that I wanted to have sex. He agreed. We got off the train at Finch station and went into the men's washroom. We were about to have sex when we noticed that I was bleeding. My monthly cycle had just started and I did not know. The guy cursed and said that he could not do it. He pulled up his pants and left. I pulled up my pants but was still horny. How could I get some sex? I decided that I would go to Jane and Finch and see if there were any opportunities.

When I got off the bus, I met a Spanish man named Victor. He was cute but was drunk. I did not know that he had been drinking. We started to talk and I told him that I wanted to have sex with him. We got off the bus at Finch and Sentinel and walked to his apartment. He lived with his parents and could not have sex there. So, went into the stairway and although I was on my period, he still had intercourse with me. It was the best sex I ever had. Days following this, we continued on this path. We had intercourse at my house many times and at the Holiday Inn close to Finch and Oakdale.

Victor and I had been spending a lot time of time together. It was like he was becoming my boyfriend and I even considered marrying him. One day, we went to liquor store to buy some Alize and beer. I had never drunk Alize before but it looked tasty, as it was blue, almost like blue Kool-Aid. We went back to my house and had sex. As a joke, I took a photo of Victor's genitals and posted it on social media. After sex, Victor decided to light up a cigarette. My landlord could smell it and came downstairs and saw us naked and yelled, *"I thought I said no smoking here. What are you doing here?"* He became irate and told him to leave. I apologized for the smoking and we left the house.

The following day, I received a few phone calls, texts, and messages about the photo I posted. They asked me to take it down. They could tell that I wasn't acting like myself but did not know what to do about it. Eventually, Facebook helped me with the picture, because they took it down for me as it was against Facebook Guidelines.

Finally, my birthday came around. The plan was to go to the restaurant inside the Trump Hotel, *The America*, for my birthday. However, a few weeks prior I made a reservation for the hotel and was unable to show because I was once again hospitalized. However, on my birthday, I invited a few friends to dinner and so far, only two people showed up, Robert and Simone. After a very hectic day, though late, I arrived to the hotel. When I arrived I was told that since I had cancelled our last dinner that I had to pay for the cost of the previous dinner. They expected me to pay approximately $800. I was shocked and asked to speak to the manager. We spoke and they said that this decision was final and we would not be able to have dinner unless I paid. Out of stress, I fainted and had a seizure. Immediately, they called the ambulance that came and attended to me. After they were done, they took me to the hospital. Both Robert and Simone came to the hospital but eventually, Robert left. I was very disappointed in him that he did not stay as years ago we were considered as best friends. However, I guess that's how life goes.

A few days later, I invited Victor with me to church. I was still manic but super happy to introduce my man to my church members. I went and introduced him to various members of the church and he really enjoyed the service. Once we were done, we went to get something to eat with one of my friends at the Swiss Chalet around the corner. We had great conversation and a great meal. Once the meal was done we went to the other side of town. We went to my old church New Life Pentecostal Church for their night service. Victor had been drinking. Considering how I was kicked out, I believed that we were there to judge the church. I sat in the back with Victor. Suddenly during service, Victor started to walk up and down the aisle. Then, he started to shout, *"No, No, No, you don't know what you're talking about"* as they were preaching. One of the brothers, the usher, came over to us and asked him to be quiet or leave. He wouldn't so I assumed that this was judgment from God for how they treated me in 2012. Finally, I got up and yelled, *"This is my church. I'm gonna come back here and buy this building and kick all of you the f**k out. Come on Victor."* I walked out the church and cursed the church that they would never grow.

Having so much sex was amazing for me. I decided to post about my experience. I wrote the following:

> *"I feel amazing! Ever since my birthday, I've been having sex again and my mental health has been so good. I know Christians are not supposed to have sex before marriage but*

I need sex. Before I became a Christian, I was a sex addict. I have been starving my body from sex and it turned into PTSD and Depression and Multiple Personality Disorder. I will be leaving for Jamaica in a few days and need your prayers. Pray that the man I am having the best sex with will marry me. I don't want to be a side chick. I want to be his main ride or die chick. I know I do not sound like I am well. You are right. I am broken. I am bruised. For now, the only drug that works for me is SEX. And, for now, I choose to keep sinning and fornicating. I don't want to fornicate but I need to in order to keep my mental health stable. Off to have more sex here at the Holiday Inn Express Toronto. #BlackAndSpanishLivesMatters."

After posting this, I received a few people who commented and prayed for me because they could see that I was going through a lot and one woman who straight out rebuked me. I did not care about the rebuke but I was grateful for the prayers.

Continuing on my sexual path, I decided to visit a few sex shops and lingerie shops, as I wanted to buy some lingerie, as I wanted to dress sexy for Victor. While shopping, I found it difficult to find my size. That's when I decided that I would come up with the idea to design lingerie for my new business, my superstore. However, I did not have a clue on how to make lingerie. I would have to find someone to make the patterns for it. Excited about my idea, I started to post photos of me showing different types of lingerie in different stores with the caption, "*Coming soon to #HappyHome42 custom made lingerie.*" Once again, I was planning something that I had no idea how to make. One day, I decided to visit my friend Dawn to tell her about my ideas. I told her about my lingerie idea and she didn't discourage but you could see that she was a bit uncomfortable with the subject. After spending a long time talking, we went to the resource centre to go to the printer. I decided to print my flyers about my lingerie company. After posting it, I handed it to a few employees at the centre, the bank and some old Italian men. I was high with excitement and continued on my path.

Victor wasn't good for me but I could not see it. I continued to have sex with him. I told him that I was broke and needed money. He showed me an illegal way that I could get money. He told me to go to the bank machine, seal an envelope, and deposit it and take out $100, as that is the minimum that banks can give you. However, he told me that I had to pay it back before the bank realized what happened. He took out $100 and gave me $80 from his account. Though I knew this was wrong, I took the money and went on my way.

Days later, I met this young man named Kevin in Ajax with his friends. I was showing them my hoodie and getting their opinion on it. I stopped them as they were going into the Best Buy. After they complimented me, I followed them into the store and continued to chat with them about my ideas and they wished me well. Kevin had mentioned that he was a fashion designer also and had a clothing line. I was very interested in seeing his work so we exchanged numbers. A few days later, I started to talk to Kevin a bit more. We became very close and he started to view me as his big sister. I would encourage him to go back to school, told him different ways that he could find money and told him I would help him with his business plan. One day we were hanging out and we wanted money. I had some cheques with me and decided I would do what Victor showed me. I had opened 4 different accounts at RBC, Scotiabank, TD bank and Bank of Montreal. So, I took my cheques and deposited it and took out $100 from each of my accounts.   Then,   I wrote a cheque to Kevin and we deposited it into his TD account and we withdrew the money right away. After that, we went out for lunch. While out, we chatted about other ways we could make money. He told me that we could take out payday loans using doctored pay stubs and bank statements. Kevin was so skilled that he was able to create both the bank statements and the bank statements. So, he created it and we went to both Cash Money and Cash For You and took out loans. I gave him half and I kept half.

Though I was doing this illegal activity, I still went to church. You see, I have never stopped going to church because I truly loved God. As I got closer to Kevin he started to tell me about his dreams and things he wanted to do in his life. I encouraged him to go back to school and was happy to hear that he was thinking about it. One day, I invited Kevin to church with me. We met up in Ajax and the first thing he noticed was my Raptors socks. He's says, *"What's up with the socks?"* I told him, *"Don't worry, its fashion."* You see when I'm manic my fashion changes. I start wearing funkier clothing. At one point I was wearing more sexual clothing. Kevin and I arrive at church and the Lord really starts to touch him, which brings him to tears. I am so excited that God is moving in his life. Due to how he felt, he decided to give his life to the Lord that day and got baptized in Jesus name. I was so happy that though people had been critical of my behavior, I still led someone to Christ.

Though still manic, I decided to continue to sleep with Victor. One night we were so horny that we decided to look for a hotel to have sex. We started in Peel and tried a Holiday Inn. They didn't accept Visa-debit cards so wouldn't let us in. I became very irate with them and they threatened that they would call the police. I dared them to call and I told them, *"Hey, I am the police!"* They called the police and I told them I would tell my social media followers to boycott their hotel. They asked me to leave the hotel and I told them that I would stay until the police came. Finally, the police arrived and they were quite hostile with us. They asked why we wouldn't leave and I told them that they are being racist and wouldn't let us in. Then, Victor, drunk with alcohol told them to f**k off and to stop bothering us. The police decided to search him while I videoed it and threatened to sue the police and the hotel. Eventually, after they found nothing they told us that we either will leave the hotel or be arrested. Determined to have sex that night, we left the hotel and found another Holiday Inn that accepted our card. We had sex all night and I was very happy.

My closest friend Dawn was becoming more and more concerned about me. I decided one night to go to her house. I had plans to go to Jamaica but I did not have a ticket. Excited that I was having sex again, I told her about my escapades and that I was finally happy. I also told her about my upcoming lingerie line. She listened to me but you could see that she was concerned. I decided to sleep at her house. I slept for a few hours and woke up around 4 am with a desire to go to Kinko's and print business cards and then go to the airport to get my ticket for Jamaica. Though I had no money for the ticket to Jamaica, I decided to go anyhow.

My mother decided to put me back in the hospital because she was frustrated with my behavior. I ended up in the Scarborough Grace General Hospital. I stayed for 11 days and due to the medication, I started to calm down from my high. When I was completely stable, I was released from the hospital and went back to my basement apartment. Once I realized what I had been doing, I decided that it was time to stop with the sexual behavior. I contacted Victor and I told him that I planned to stop seeing him. He was disappointed but he agreed.

Chapter 14:
Babies are Blessings

Though I loved my basement apartment, I longed for an apartment where I could get sunshine. Finally, after approximately two years of waiting I was approved for subsidized housing five minutes away from my CMHA Act Team's office. I was truly excited. I told my landlord's that I would be moving and though disappointed they understood. I started to pack my things and moved into my apartment for June 1st, 2016. Excited about the move, I told my friends that I would plan a housewarming party when I settled in. I continued to talk to my friend Kevin about fashion and going back to school. I even told him that I looked forward to having him come over for dinner. We looked forward to this. Weeks later Kevin was tragically murdered and was found in front of his building. I was shocked and truly saddened by this event. Filled with grief, I went to the funeral to pay my final respects. Though I was saddened, I believed he was in a better place.

Motivated to start my fashion business, I decided to start sewing again. I would sew African inspired clothing for myself and determined that I would become a designer that made custom made skirts for women. Though motivated, I slowly started to become manic again. I started to brainstorm ideas on how I could expand my business and came up with the idea to sell gift cards. I went to Kinko's and printed these paper gift cards and tried to sell them.

One night while full blown manic, I met a young man named Steven. I offered him an opportunity to join my business and he was intrigued. We went into a Burger King and started to talk about the gift cards. He liked the idea and I told him that I didn't want the night to end. Being close to my home, we decided to walk and talk. I followed him to his home and went down into his basement apartment. He was a renting a bedroom in the basement and it was so dirty. I was not impressed. Although unimpressed, we started to talk and I asked him if he wanted to come to my apartment to watch a movie or something. He agreed. With only a 15-minute walk to my house, we decided to walk to my home. As we walked, he started to smoke his cigarettes and marijuana. He offered me a cigarette and I took one even though I didn't smoke. However, that night, I was a smoker. Finally, we arrived at my apartment. We continued to talk and then watched a movie. At the end of the movie, I told him he could sleep on my sofa while I would sleep on my bed. I got undressed for bed and went into my bed when I saw him at the door. He slipped into my bed, and said he wanted to lie beside me. I allowed him to lie down beside me and I started to drift off to sleep. In my drowsy state, he started to kiss my neck slowly and gently. I hadn't had sex since Victor and was aware of becoming nervous. As he continued to kiss me, I started to loosen up. Eventually, we had sex that night.

As the days passed by, we started to see each other every day. I would take selfies with him and go with him to various places to try to sell my gift cards. Every day for about two weeks, we would meet up and have sex at my apartment. After the 3rd day, I asked him if I could call him my boyfriend. He agreed. I was elated. I had a real boyfriend. I felt special but I was still manic. Finally, at the end of the two weeks, I started to notice he had some bad habits. He was either always drinking or high on marijuana. He also had a temper. As one day, I was combing his hair and he called me names because he said I was combing his hair too hard. I was pissed and started to come down from my high and started to notice to see his flaws. The more I saw his flaws, the more I disliked him. At the end of the 2nd week, I decided that it was time to end our relationship. I called Steven and told him that I did not want to see him again. However, during our time together, we had unprotected sex once.

It had been about a month and my period hadn't come yet. I was nervous as I forgot to go to the clinic and get the plan B pill the night I had unprotected sex. Fearful of being pregnant, I called two friends and told them that I might be pregnant. They asked me if I took a pregnancy test. I told them that I didn't take one yet. Melinda, one of my friends, told me that the dollar store had pregnancy tests. She also told me that I should get a blood test to make sure. So, I went to the dollar store and bought the pregnancy test. When I arrived home, I took the test and when I saw the result I started to cry. I couldn't believe that I was pregnant. Since, I was not convinced, I went to my doctor and got a blood test. A few days later, I went back to get the results and it was confirmed. I was pregnant. Cleoni Crawford was pregnant.

I called three of my girlfriends Dawn, Melinda and Corrine about my ordeal. Each woman gave me different advice but I was determined to have an abortion. I was not gonna have this baby. I was not ready to have a child. Having a child was not in the cards for me. My mental illness was too sporadic and I feared that I could not be a good mother. All three women encouraged me to keep the child. Dawn referred me to a place called the Pregnancy Care Centre to talk about my options for pregnancy. She said that they helped her when she was pregnant. My other friend, Melinda told me she would support me despite my decision.

I felt good knowing that I wouldn't be judged for my decision to have this abortion. The following day, I decided to tell my CMHA worker Maisha that I was pregnant. They were very supportive and listened to me. I told them that I was considering an abortion. Upon hearing this, they told me they would support me despite my decision. However, my psychiatrist at the time, Dr. Johnston, recommended that I had the abortion considering my mental health. As I was about to leave, the occupational therapist, handed me a pamphlet for the Pregnancy Care Centre. I looked at it and said, *"I guess I really need to visit this place as my friend also told me about it."*

The following day, I contacted the Pregnancy Care Centre to make an appointment to see a counselor. They accepted me and later that day I went to the Scarborough location, as that was the closest to me. When I arrived at the address, I noticed that they were inside a church, the Morningstar Fellowship church. I knocked on the door and out came a beautiful black woman. She introduced herself as Paulette and led me into a cozy room with a sofa. She gave me some forms to fill out about my pregnancy for the assessment. When I got to the part about the father, I couldn't answer many of the questions such as his date of birth or even address. I remember feeling quite embarrassed that I did not know enough about this man. Once completed, Paulette re-entered the room and we began to talk. We talked about how I got pregnant and the involvement of the father. I mentioned that he was denying the baby and that I just needed an abortion. They told me that I had three options: to parent, to put up for adoption or to abort. They explained each option. The first option they discussed was to parent. They talked about all the programs they had to support the parent and how possible it was. Then they talked about abortion by explaining what the procedure looked like. As they explained it, I started to feel uncomfortable in my vagina. They said it wouldn't hurt much but it was like a vacuum. Finally, they discussed the adoption process. Once they were done explaining my options, I asked if they could provide any recommendations for abortion clinics because I just wanted to get rid of the baby, they told me that due to the type of clinic they were, they could not provide such a list and I would have to look it up independently. At the close of the meeting, they closed in prayer and I went home.

Despite the opinions, I decided that I was going to have an abortion. I pulled out my computer and started to search for abortion clinics in Google. After searching, I found a list of clinics in Toronto that I could attend. After reading through the website and checking the reviews of each clinic, I decided on two clinics: The Bay street clinic and the Morgentaler clinic. Immediately, I contacted both clinics and made appointment for later that week on a Thursday and the other on the following Monday. After making the appointments, I felt a sigh of relief. The following day, a new friend of mine, Laure contacted me and I told her that I was pregnant. She was not judgmental towards me. She told me the story of her children and encouraged me to keep the baby. I told her that I could not keep the child and that I was going to have an abortion. She asked if I would meet her before I attended my appointment at the Morgentaler abortion clinic. I agreed. The following day, she picked me up and took me to her church in Ajax where I met her pastor. The three of us opened up in prayer and we started to chat. While talking about my pregnancy, the pastor said, *"Please do not kill that baby. The bible says 'Before I formed the in the belly I knew thee; and before thou camest forth out of the womb I sanctified thee.' What that* means is that God knows about your baby as a fetus. Your baby is already a living soul." When he said that, for the first time ever since pregnant, I was convicted about this baby. This baby was no longer just a baby but actually a living soul. With that revelation, I made the decision that I would carry the baby to term but give it up for adoption. When I went home that afternoon, I called the Morgentaler and the Bay street clinic and cancelled my appointments.

Now that I decided that I would keep the baby, I decided that it was time to share this information with my Pastor. I made an appointment to see the Pastor. Eventually, the date came and I went to church to see my Pastor, Pastor Castro. We opened up in prayer and then I shared that I was pregnant. You could see that he was disappointed but was more worried that disappointed. I told him that I was considering giving the child up for adoption. He thought that would be a good option and offered to provide as much support as possible. I left the meeting feeling relieved and supported. As I was leaving, I saw a sister who asked me how I was doing, I blurted out, *"I'm pregnant."* She looked at me in shock and disgust. You could see the disappointment in her face. She was not happy about this and was pretty negative about it. Despite this, I ignored her reaction and kept it moving. Later that day, I spoke to my friend Corinne and told her about my discussion with the Pastor and how well it went. She was thankful. I also told her about that sister's reaction and she told me that I should have never told her because she is a chatterbox and now everyone was going to know about my pregnancy. I regretted telling that sister but I didn't let that bother me.

I called Steven, the father of the baby, to tell him that I was pregnant and was having his baby. He denied it all the way.

He called me a whore and a liar. He said I was trying to trap him into having this baby. We yelled back and forth and he told me to go and find the father of this baby, as it was not his. I was so upset so I hung up the phone to calm down. Sadly, it went on like this for a few months, where he continued to deny this baby.

Now that I decided to put the child up for adoption, I went back to my CMHA office and met my psychiatrist again. I told him that I was not going to have the abortion. He told me that I was making the worst decision in my life. He continued that choosing to keep this baby would ruin my life and I needed to reconsider. I was so disappointed in my doctor and couldn't believe how hostile he had become. I left his office upset and asked to speak with Maisha from the team. I told her what the doctor said and she was shocked but offered words to comfort me. I felt much better after talking to her. I left the office and went home.

A few months had passed and I was getting bigger and bigger. This pregnancy was getting more and more real by the moment. However, I was still determined to give my baby up for adoption. One day while in conversation with my mother, I reminded her that I would be giving my child up for adoption. In frustration, my mother abruptly said, "*If anything happens, I will take the baby for you.*" When I heard this, I now felt as though I truly had the support I needed to raise the baby. With that said, I made the decision then and there that I was going to parent and keep my baby. A few days later, I made an appointment with the Pregnancy Care Centre to share my news. When Paulette at the Pregnancy Care Centre heard that I had decided to parent, she was so excited. She told me about the Life Boat program and recommended I take the course, as it would prepare me for raising my child. It was a 4-week course, and helps parents plan for the birth of their baby. It includes such topics such as making good decisions, realities of parenting and financial budgeting. It was a really great program as it opened my mind up to the things that I would have to prepare for like the cost of having a baby. At the end of the financial planning part, I remember feeling very defeated and depressed because I did not have the money to buy all the things that my child would need. However, after speaking to a friend, she encouraged me and said, *"Babies bring blessings."* She also told me that whatever my needs were that God would work it out and open doors. Though I had a hard time believing this, months later, I got to see the saying "*babies bring blessings*" come to pass.

When I became pregnant, I was taking two types of medications: one for my bipolar and the other for my epilepsy. One of my fears was that I would need to stop taking my medication and would in turn become sick again. That scared me. The other thing I feared was how my medication would affect my child should I continue to take it. After an appointment with my doctor, I was told that my epilepsy medication could cause my child to have cleft lip. I was very concerned about my child having any birth defects. Another thing that I was concerned about is my child having Down syndrome. Though I knew that it would not be the end of the world, I really wanted a healthy baby. If God allowed me to have a baby with birth defects, I would consider that God was punishing me. I did not want my child to have to go through half of what I went through with my illnesses. I just wanted him or her to be healthy. Due to these fears, my monthly appointments with my gynecologist were not pleasant. At each appointment, I went in there fearful that I would receive some bad news about my child's progress. Though I would get the chance to hear the heart beat or see the baby growing inside of me, I was very fearful that something would be wrong. My OB appointments were more stressful than they were joyful. The only appointment that I was happy to go to was when they revealed the sex of the baby. I was praying for a boy and did not want a girl. Thankfully, God granted me my wish. I was having a baby boy.

As it grew closer and closer to my due date, I started to think about all the people I had offended and questioned if anyone would attend my baby shower if I had one. When I was manic, I had offended so many people that I thought I did not have any friends left. I believed that I wouldn't have anyone that would help me with my baby outside my family and close friends. Boy was I wrong. My baby sister Feleisha planned my baby shower for me and I was so shocked by the amount of people who showed up and the gifts I received. With the help of the Pregnancy Care Centre, the attendees of my shower, and complete strangers, I received a new stroller with car seat, crib, bouncer, playpen, high chair, seven garbage bags of clothing and 40 pairs of shoes for my son. I was truly blessed because babies did indeed bring blessings. I could not believe that there were so many people that cared about my son and I.

My due date was just around the corner; it was for April 27th, 2017. A few weeks before my due date, my doctor noticed that my blood pressure was getting higher. After the 2nd week of seeing my blood pressure so high, she decided that she was going to schedule me to be induced two days before my actual due date. I was quite nervous but prepared. I had prepared a small suitcase of clothing to wear while in the hospital. Due to my mental illness, I was going to be in the hospital for five days so they could assess my ability to parent. While in the hospital, I was to meet a social
worker and a psychiatrist who would monitor me to make sure that I could raise my son without any complications. Finally, the date

came for me to be induced. I had my mother pick me up and we went to Scarborough Grace Hospital. My labour took a very long time. They had given me Pitocin through an IV and catheters to help me go into labour over a span of two days to no success. After two days of labour, my cervix only dilated to 6 cm. The staff decided that they were going to do the scheduled C-section.

Finally, at 8:13 am, my baby boy, Emmanuel Gabriel Crawford was born. I remember when I woke up from the C-section, they showed me my baby and I felt so overjoyed. I've never felt such joy. It was an amazing feeling.

Once the surgery was done, they wheeled me into my room where I waited with my mother for my new baby boy to return. When the nurse came in with my son, I gasped, as he was so precious. He had big beautiful eyes with the longest eyelashes ever. He was absolutely perfect and I was thankful for him. He had his 10 toes, 10 fingers, two eyes, one nose, one mouth and one huge belly button. He was mine and I was so happy. As normal, I posted a photo of my son on WhatsApp and Facebook and received many comments. As the comments came in, so came the visitors. I had so many people come to visit us in the hospital. The support I was received was phenomenal. Everyone kept mentioning how cute my son was. I was a proud mommy. Of the many visitors, my godmother, Marcia came to visit me. Since she was not working, she offered to come and help me with the baby while I recovered. Considering that I was a new mother and I knew my mother could only help for two weeks, I told her I would take her up on her offer.

Since I became pregnant, I had no manic episodes. This was the longest that I had been healthy with no manic episodes in years. That was a miracle. With this miracle, I had to prove to the doctors and social worker that I was able to take care of my son without any concerns. Considering that the hospital staff was monitoring me, I was extra cautious. In order to ensure that the doctors were satisfied with my behavior, my mother stayed with me for the whole five days at the hospital. While there, I would constantly pray over my son and for myself that God will grant me favour in the eyes of my doctors and my social worker. Finally, the psychiatrist came to evaluate me. He asked me many questions about my mood and I answered them to his liking. A day later, the social worker came and asked me questions. Thankfully, I was able to answer the questions to his liking as well. Finally, the 5th day came and it was time to hear back from the psychiatrist and get clearance to go home. He arrived and gave me clearance to go home, as they had no concerns about my ability to take care of my child. I was ecstatic. Once I was received the clearance, I got my son ready in his clothing and we left the hospital in his new car seat.

I was relieved to be home; however, I no longer had nurses watching my son as I slept. Now it was time to get to business. I was a mother and I had to be the one who woke up at nights to feed my son. It was hard at first but I managed. Since I had a C-section, I had to heal from my cut and also needed to get a lot of sleep. At first, my mother stayed with me for another week. Then, I received help from an organization named VHA. They provided a free PSW that would come to my house 3 mornings a week. She would watch my son while I slept. I remember being so tired every morning from being woken up every few hours to feed my son at night that as soon as my PSW came, I would just hand the baby to her as soon as she took her shoes off. I looked forward to seeing her, as she was such a blessing. This PSW provided help for 3 months. It was amazing. The second help I received was from my godmother Marcia. She came Tuesdays and Thursdays to help me take care of Emmanuel. She was such a blessing, as she would stay for most of the day. Since I was still healing, she would also help me cook. Also, a few members of my church came a few nights to sleep over to help me handle the nights. Nights were the most challenging but over time, I started to get used to waking up so many times.

Finally, my son's father was starting to believe that he might in fact have a son. I had been requesting his mother's number because I wanted her to know that she had a grandson. After many months of asking, he gave me her number. Her name was Grace. It was Mother's Day and I called her up and introduced myself to her and told her that she had a grandson and his name was Emmanuel. She was so happy to hear that but wanted to see a photo of the child to make sure it was his. I sent her a photo via WhatsApp and she was convinced immediately as my son looks exactly like him.

Since then, she's been a very important part of our lives. She scheduled a visit to come and see the baby with her two sons Danique and Dante. They came over and they instantly fell in love with my son.

Chapter 15:
Manic

It had been six weeks since my son was born and I really missed being at church. However, I wasn't going back to church until I healed and my son got christened. So, on June 11, 2017, I returned back to church for my son's baby dedication. I bought him this three-piece suit with a lovely bow tie. He was so cute. I invited my family and friends over to the dedication and it was well attended. The only person that did not attend was his father. However, by the end of the dedication, my son pooped up the whole leg of his pants. Thankfully, I had already taken my photos with him in the suit so we just changed him. At the end of the service, some of us went to a Jamaican restaurant in Pickering for dinner. It was just under 20 of us there and we had a great time.

It had been 3 months since my son was born and I decided to put him into daycare as I was going to go to school in September. As a woman who was on disability, I qualified to have my son in subsidized daycare for free whether or not I was working or attending school. I was given the chance to get relief support for him as long as I was on disability. Thankfully, the daycare was located downstairs in the building. This made it convenient for me as I didn't have to worry about taking my son on the bus to get to daycare. I remember the first day I brought him there, he didn't cry but I cried on my way out. Thankfully, my son was in great care. The women, Nicola, Yvonne and Allison were so good to him. He was the youngest baby there and they took really good care of him.

It had been a whole year since I was manic and people were so proud of me. People from church and abroad would tell me how proud they were of me and how much of a good mother I was. I was thankful that I had remained stable for so long. The Pregnancy Care Centre asked me if I would do an interview about my progress and I agreed. With my son in hand, we recorded the interview. I discussed my mental health, how much they helped me and how I almost aborted my son. By the end of the interview, the interviewer mentioned how inspired they were of me. We took photos and called it a day.

I had decided that it was time to go back to school to finish my fashion program at George Brown College. So I re-registered and started in September. Since I still had outstanding loans from OSAP, I did not qualify for any loans and had to pay it myself. With the help of my mother, we paid for my first semester of school. I was so excited to be back in school doing what I loved, though I was only able to handle part time studies. I took my core subjects of sewing, drafting, and technical illustration; still, I had a lot of homework and it was intense. I was constantly doing homework. Thankfully, I had my neighbor Margaret help by picking up my son a few nights a week and keeping him till I got home. I do not know how I would have done it without her.

The Pregnancy Care Centre was so pleased with my interview in the summer that they decided that they would play my video at their annual fundraising dinner. I was ecstatic. Also, to promote the dinner, they requested that I go on the radio with them with two other women, my friends Dawn and Angie. I agreed and was really looking forward to sharing my story with the masses. The show was going to be on WDCX radio and was going on live. It had been a while since I had been on the radio and I was a bit nervous but excited. I made a post promoting the interview on my social media pages in hopes of getting my supporters to listen in. Once again, people were so proud of me and said they would listen. Finally, it came time for the interview and though nervous, I did a great job. After the interview, people contacted me congratulating me. I was truly proud of myself and thankful. A few days later, I posted the interview I did in the summer with the Pregnancy Care Centre on my social media and on the Black Moms Connection group and received a lot of feedback. People mentioned how inspired they were of me. With all of this attention, I was feeling good and proud of my accomplishments.

A few weeks later, it was time for the Pregnancy Care Centre annual fundraising dinner and I was dressed in a gown and looked like a princess. My son was dressed in a three-piece suit. Together, we looked as though we were ready for a ball. It was a really great event. They showed my video and then called me up on the stage with my son. I was excited to be up there as I had been doing so well. Life was looking good for me.

It had been a few months since I had joined the Facebook group the Black Moms Connection. They had become my village of support. Whenever I would post in the group, I would get a lot of likes and support. I simply loved the group and was so grateful for them. On December 2, 2017, I decided to post some sketches I did for an assignment and received so much positive feedback. In total, I had received 452 likes and 231 comments praising my work.

One of those likes was from a Member of Parliament from Whitby who also suffered with depression. I was inspired by her story. Under my photo, she mentioned that she would purchase my stuff once I started my business and I was ecstatic. With that comment, I decided that I would make a gown for her at my fashion show that I was going to host the following year when I graduated. Though I said this, I still did not know how to make gowns. However, I was going to be taking the bridal and evening gowns course for the following semester so I was making this comment by faith. I decided to send her a private message telling her about this and she liked the idea. I also requested to schedule a meet and greet and she agreed for a meeting in January. I was so excited. Life was looking good.

However, later that month, things started to take a turn for the worse. One morning I woke up really early and decided that I would think of a way that I could raise money for school for my second semester. I came up with the idea to create a website called Help Me Finish Fashion School and created a GoFundMe page. I made of a video of me sitting in front of my sewing machine requesting for financial help with school. I posted this hyperlink everywhere online. Some people were supportive and some people were quite hostile. Some people thought that I shouldn't be begging money for school and that it was inappropriate. Despite what people thought, I kept posting. Though my posts were focused at first, they started to become spammy. I started to post my hyperlink in everything I posted and would tag at least 50 people in each post including the MP. I didn't realize it but I was becoming manic again. I would tag her in everything. To me, I wasn't being spammy but when I look back at the posts, I realize I was.

I started to get calls from a friend of mine Corrine who was concerned about my posts. She noticed that I had been posting a lot and wanted to make sure that I was alright. However, I took it as though she was trying to stop me and became very critical of her. I was feeling as though people like Corrine were against me.

Due to amount of negative attention I was getting, I was starting to have anxiety attacks. My chest would start to hurt me and I would have trouble breathing. I remember one day I was trying to calm myself down by listening to music and then Corrine called, starting to judge me based on my posts. I hung up the phone on her. She kept calling back so I kept declining her calls. Then, she sent me a voice note on WhatsApp that sounded as though she was trying to boss me around.

I was highly offended and irritable. Immediately after that, I left my house and went to my CMHA office to talk about what I was going through. I spoke to my worker Angela and played the voice note to her and she understood why I was feeling the way I was. I told Angela that I was stressed out by my friend Corrine and I wanted her friendship but she was causing me to have anxiety attacks. I simply wanted her to relax. So, Angela called Corrine on speaker and spoke to her while I listened. She tried to explain what mental illness looked like, how to be supportive and that I was fine. She disagreed with her and told her that she believed that I was manic and needed help. I was very angry and rebutted her comments and then we hung up the phone. Though I was critical of Corrine, I know now that she was trying to help the best way she knew how.

After the meeting I calmed down and went home. However, once there I was still upset and started to have an anxiety attack so I called my son's grandmother Grace crying. I begged her to take my son because I wasn't doing well. She agreed and picked him up from daycare. The following day, I decided to go downtown and Corrine called me to check up on me. I told her that I was taking a walk downtown and she was okay with my response. I hung up the phone annoyed by her. The following day was church and my son was still visiting his paternal grandmother Grace for the weekend, so I was free for the weekend. I went church and told people that I was being stressed out by Corrine and that she was causing me to have anxiety attacks. She was there and became upset about that and pushed me as I was in the coatroom and I snapped. We started cursing each other. One of the ushers, Brother Richard stepped up and took me home. While in the car, I started to disgrace her and call her all kinds of names. I slut shamed her in front of Richard and he had no words. By the time I arrived at home, I was so angry and that I decided that I was going to disgrace her online. I started to post intimate details about her and slut shamed her online for hours. I started to say that the death angel was coming to kill her. In addition, I put her address online and told people that they could have sex with her. I posted about her all night long and did not sleep. When I think it over, I was very wrong and should not have dragged her in the mud like I did. However, when I'm manic I can be very nasty and rude.

By the time it was morning, I was exhausted and a complete mess. Suddenly, I started to feel fearful and did not want to leave my house. My house was a complete mess. There were papers everywhere and I had not combed nor desired to comb my hair. Usually on Mondays, Wednesdays and Fridays I see someone from the ACT team. Today being Monday, I was supposed to go to the office for my routine visit. However, I simply couldn't leave my house and asked if they would do a home visit instead. One of the reps came and we talked. She suggested that I see my psychiatrist, Dr. Ferguson, immediately the following day. I agreed. Once she left, I called my neighbor, Margaret and asked her if she would come to my apartment. I started to cry and told her that I was not doing well and needed her to take my son and take care of him until I got better. Additionally, I asked her to attend my appointment with me the following day and she agreed to both requests. She gathered some clothing from me and left.

The following morning, I got ready to see my psychiatrist. I decided to wear one of my long dresses, as I did not want to be seen as that I was unwell. However, there was a lot of snow outside, so this was a bad choice. I did not want to be hospitalized but simply wanted some medication to help me calm down. When I arrived at the appointment, I was frustrated with everyone including white doctors. I told her I wanted to speak to Dr. Kwame McKenzie, a black well-known psychiatrist. Recently, I had met him at a conference and he talked about how many doctors misdiagnose and don't acknowledge that some people have PTSD. I believed that I had PTSD along with my bipolar but wanted to be treated for the trauma I had experienced. She didn't agree and after speaking to my sister, my friend Terry from Atlanta and my father, she made the decision that she was going to have me hospitalized. Although I asked for some medication to calm me down, she told me to go into the conference room and she would be right back. After waiting in the small conference room with my neighbor Margaret, suddenly two police officers came. They were there to take me to the hospital as my doctor was putting me on form 1 for psychiatric evaluation. I was extremely upset about this but eventually after yelling that I was going to sue left the office with the officers.

I had carried my iPad, iPhone and MacBook with me to the hospital. Along the way, I was listening to my music to keep me calm. I would sing and dance in the waiting room. Then, the nurses came to take away my devices and I became so upset that I started throwing things and hurling insults at them. I threw the mattress off the bed and tried to throw other things but most of the other things were nailed down. I started to bang on the window, *"Give me my phone, give me my f**king phone!"* Eventually, the nurse came in the room with two security officers and I knew exactly what that meant. I resisted and they strapped me down to the bed and gave me a needle. I lay on the bed and started to cry. Hours later, my godmother, Marcia came to the hospital and saw me strapped to the bed. She was saddened to see me like this. I told her that I was hungry so she left and got me something to eat and fed me since I couldn't feed myself. Apparently the doctors had contacted Children's Aid since they found out that I was a mother. I did not know this until later. I only spent the minimum 3 days or 72 hours in the Centenary hospital and then was released.

After being released I came down from my high and was no longer manic. However, I was sorrowful to how I treated my friend Corrine. I realized that I should not have disgraced her the way I did. Though regretful, I had two appointments that I was looking forward to attending: my healing retreat with Ellel Ministries and my appointment with the MP from Whitby. Though excited, the meeting with the MP did not go as I hoped. I started off by thanking her for meeting me and started showing some of sketches. I told her what type of dress I would like to make for her. She told me that she couldn't accept a gift that extravagant. I asked if she would be willing to purchase such a gift and she said she hadn't seen my stitching skills. Then, told her more about the fashion show that I wanted to plan with her office. She asked me how much I had planned and I told her that I wanted to plan it with her office and she said that usually when people see her that they usually have their events already planned. Finally, I asked if I could have a photo with her and she declined and this is when she told me that she felt harassed by me. She said that the multiple tags felt like harassment. I did not realize this but when I look back and try to see it from her perspective, I can see why she felt harassed. This was the first time that I started to see how my multiple tags to people could be seen as harassment or bothersome. At the end of the meeting, I left feeling quite disappointed.

Though saddened, I cheered myself up with the realization that I would be going to Westport Ontario, north of Kingston Ontario, to the Ellel Ministries Healing Retreat. I was told about this place as being a place where you could get delivered from your illnesses. I no longer wanted to have my illness hold me down again.

That healing retreat was such a blessing to me. I learned so much about myself and my family line that it was shocking. In a nutshell, I learned that there were 23 different spirits that were affecting my family line of which 9 were affecting me personally. Specifically, this is what they found in my generational line: anger, bitterness, adultery, addiction, sexual sin, rejection, divorce, fornication, witchcraft/occult/hexing, superstition, mental illness, gossip, abandonment, abortion, blood sacrifice, yoga, jezebel, Alzheimer, Schizophrenia, Bipolar, Infirmity, madness and death. When I saw this list I was shocked and couldn't believe that there were so many issues in my family. However, it started to make sense why I was going through so much in my life. To me, I always knew that my mental illness was not just chemical but spiritual. I believed that both aspects were affecting me. When I left the retreat, I started to post my testimony on social media. I was so thankful that we were able to pray and cancel its assignment on my life. Though we prayed, I knew it was a process. It would never end in one day but over time.

Since I started to share my testimony online I found this woman named Simone who had an organization called Essence of Mind that was hosting an event called Black Trauma for Black History Month. She made a post about trauma and I responded that I had experienced my own trauma. From there, we started to chat and she asked if I would be willing to share my story at her event. I was excited to be asked and started to promote her event on my social media pages and abroad. However, though I was excited about the event, I was becoming more and more manic by the day. I started to post constantly and become hostile and judgmental. I would post about judgment on people in politics that weren't acting right. I even posted about Donald Trump losing his life or his job by a specific date. I was very specific with the dates. From the outside looking in, they could see that I was unwell, but in my eyes I was moving into my calling as a prophetess again. It was my job to see the sins of the world and judge them. I was becoming grandiose in my thinking.

While posting, I decided to tag the MP again and was reprimanded by her. She responded, *"I thought we talked about this!"* in an angry tone. At the moment, it was like something snapped because I started to tell her that I was a prophetess and that she was going to be judged for her mistreatment of me. I started to post that if she didn't donate money to my cause by a specific date that she would receive judgement and even death. This scared her so much that she decided to contact the police. The officer that called me knew about my mental illness and was very calm with me. He explained that I needed to stop posting about her because she felt harassed. However, despite this call, I felt like I couldn't stop. I became obsessed and couldn't explain why. Then, the police called again and said they wanted to meet me at my house to hand me some documents. At first, I told them that I would meet them there and then I heard a voice that said, *"They are coming to arrest you."* With that said, I told myself that I would leave the country.

I went to the Toronto Pearson airport and tried to get a flight to Jamaica with no money. My thoughts were that I would use the credit that was applied to my friend Terry's ticket that I had bought in December. When that didn't work, I decided I would call my father and see if he would give me the money. Instead, he yelled at me and told me that he was going to tell the police where to find me. About 30 minutes later, I saw the police in the airport and assumed that they were there to find me. I became so fearful that they were after me, so I kept walking back and forward and then mustered up the courage to walk pass them and wave at them as well. They smiled at me and then I left the airport and said I would leave the province and go to my second home, Montreal.

When I left the airport, I decided to call my cousin Shay and see if she could loan me $50 to cover the cost to pay for my ticket to Montreal. She didn't have the money but her sister did and said that I could have it. However, in order to get it, I had to come and see her. So, I went on the bus and to Armel court I went. I finally arrived and was really cold and needed more comfortable shoes. I went into the building, knocked the door but they weren't home at the moment, so I waited in the hallway. After about 30 minutes, they arrived. I went inside their home and we talked about many different spiritual forces that were affecting our families while eating dinner. At the end, her sister, Kelly, went online and purchased my ticket to Montreal. Then, Shay gave me a pair of shoes, winter jacket and scarf that I could use as I was cold an on my way to Montreal. They then drove me to the nearest subway station and set me on my way.

I arrived at the Toronto Bus terminal on Bay St. and waited for my bus. Then, I saw the police in front of the terminal and questioned within myself if they were looking for me. Since I had been posting many selfies of myself wearing certain clothing, I decided to use my scarf to cover my head like a hijab and waited in the line for the bus. I turned off the data on all my devices just in case they were tracking my phone. Finally my bus arrived and I stood in line waiting to show my ticket to the bus driver. I was so fearful that the police might have found me and tried to have me arrested. Thankfully, though only several feet away from the police, I was able to board the bus undetected.

En route to Montreal, I made sure that I turned off my phone just in case the police was tracking me. While on the bus, to keep me entertained, I turned on my computer and watched movies and slept. Before I arrived in Montreal, I knew that I needed a place to stay and decided that I wanted to stay at the most expensive hotel in the city, the Fairmont Queen Elizabeth Hotel. I gave them a call and made a reservation.

Hours later, approximately 2:30pm, I arrived in Montreal and proceeded to walk to the hotel since I did not have any money. Though I did not have money, I knew that I could possibly show them my credit card and if it didn't go through, I could stay there till morning at least. When I arrived at the hotel, I went to the desk and showed them my President's Club rewards card and they found my booking. They asked for my credit card and I showed them my prepaid card. Unfortunately, they didn't accept it but said they would take the full payment for three nights on my debit card. Knowing that it wouldn't go through, I gave them my card just for show. Surprisingly, the transaction went through for over $800. I was shocked because I knew there was no money in the account but I acted like everything was normal. They gave me my key and I went up to my room.

I was so excited that I, queen and prophetess, was staying at the most prestigious hotel in the city. While there, I decided that I would create a new Instagram called Queenfoo42 and then I simply changed it to Queen42inc, as it sounded more professional. I also told people to call me by my new name Queen Crawford, because I was a Queen staying in the Queen's hotel. In my eyes, I was a new woman.

The following morning, I decided it was time to go site seeing and find out where the Adidas head office was. I found out that it was outside the city off a highway. I found the instructions and made plans to go there on the 31st of January when I received money. In the meantime, I travelled around the city. I would post on social media that I was in Montreal and having a blast. Though I posted about the different places I had been, I would not post about where I was staying, just in case the police in Montreal was following me too. Then I received a phone call from the police in Ontario saying that they were disappointed that I did not show up to my apartment that night. I told them I was on a vacation and would see them when I got back. I hung up the phone. The second call I received was from Simone from Essence of Mind about the event Black Trauma. Due to my previous negative social media activity, she was disinviting me to speak at her event. She didn't want all the negative attention that I was getting. I was disappointed but I understood.

Once I finished my call, I realized that I needed a lawyer. So, I contacted a well-known law firm in Montreal and posted that I would be going there for legal advice. When I was almost there, I saw about five police cars surrounding the law firm. This is when I realized that the Montreal police were after me too. So, I turned and went in the opposite direction. When I was far enough away, I made a post saying that I would not be using that law firm anymore and mocked the police for thinking I was stupid. I then, continued to walk and seek out another lawyer. I made a few calls and finally found a lawyer via phone. I told her that I think I might be in trouble with the law in Ontario and wanted advice as to what to do. She gave me advice and I decided to return back to my hotel.

When I went back to the hotel, I called my good friend Terry from Atlanta and we had a long conversation. We joked around and I told him that I couldn't wait to see him in Canada. I told him that

I was going to go to Jamaica first to get the denim dress I made in class mass-produced. Once again, I did not have the money to mass produce anything but knew that I would get the money in a loan. I wanted to use Jamaica because I wanted to give back to my people and not use China. After talking about everything under the sun, I went to bed and called it a night.

Chapter 16:
Finding Purpose

While I was in Montreal my son was still at my neighbor/babysitter/godmother's house. I knew that he was well taken care of, as she absolutely adored my son. However, at that time, I was in no position to take care of my son. Knowing this, I left him in her care. I didn't realize how long it had been because of all the things I was up to. Then, one day while still in the hotel, I receive a phone call from a woman named Natalie from Children's Aid. The previous month, we had met with a worker and it was determined that all was fine. However, with me gone for so long, they decided that they were going to put my son under a kinship agreement. That meant that my son was going to be under the care of Margaret until Children's Aid determined that I could care for him again. At first, I agreed to it but did not realize the long-term effects of this arrangement. Natalie was simply calling me as a courtesy to let me know that this was happening.

The following morning, I woke up very early because something didn't feel right. With this feeling, I decided I would leave the hotel very early in the morning around 4 am. Before I left the hotel, I took a photo of myself in front of the Queen Elizabeth hotel plaque and posted how thankful I was for them being so hospitable to me. I mentioned how much of a great hotel they were and left. I walked for about an hour and then became quite leery when I saw police cars. I remember walking towards one and going the opposite direction to avoid it. I finally arrived at the bus stop to go to the Adidas head office. My plan was to go there and talk about a partnership with them and then go straight to the airport for Jamaica. I waited about 30 minutes for my bus in the nearby McDonalds, as it was freezing cold.

When my bus arrived, I travelled along the highway towards my destination and then, the transit police came on the bus and asked for my pass. I showed it to them but was so fearful because I thought they were looking for me. They then left the bus and I left the bus as well as I had discovered that I missed my stop. I crossed the street to wait for the next bus. While standing at the bus stop, I called my friend Trish and asked for a favour. I asked her to loan me the money to buy my ticket for Jamaica until my next pay. She agreed and we talked on the phone while I waited for the bus. Then, the transit police drove to where I was standing for the bus. I thought they were following me and then after 20 minutes they drove off. Finally, my bus arrived and I got off at my stop. The weather was horrible and freezing cold.

It was too early to go to the Adidas Head Office as it was still closed so I went into a hotel nearby. Frost bitten, I requested a room so I could sleep in for a few hours and they gave me one for $80. I was pissed that it was so expensive for only two hours but that was the policy. So, I went into my room, took a shower, bought my ticket to Jamaica online and took a nap. When I woke up, I checked out and walked over to the Adidas Head Office. When I arrived, I discovered that the Montreal location had closed down most of their operations and transferred it to Toronto. I could not believe that I came all that way just to find out that they weren't there.

Disappointed, I left the Adidas Head office, called a taxi and went straight to the airport for my flight.

When I arrived at the airport, I went through customs, showed them my ticket and proceeded to the gate for Jamaica. I was so excited to be going to Jamaica. I had plans to create business relationships for my fashion business and was super excited. Then, as it was time to board the plan, the airport police tapped me on the shoulder and called me by name and said, *"Excuse me Ms. Crawford."* I responded. Then, they told me that there was a Canada-wide warrant out for my arrest for uttering threats. I became angry as this was the second time that I was prevented from going to Jamaica. I asked them if they were preventing me from going on my flight and they said yes. I took to social media and started to post about this and how outraged I was and uttered another death threat, which said, *"that b***h called the police on me. I don't care, shottas, shoot up her whole family."* Please note, I have no shottas or have ever had a gun. I was just angry that this MP was preventing me from doing business in Jamaica.

The officers took me to a back room and started to explain why I was being prevented from travelling and that the Ontario police would be coming to bring me back to Ontario. Though pissed, I was cooperative. They took me to jail and I stayed in the cell for the whole day. It was freezing and I was hungry. They gave me two box juices and two breakfast bars to eat. I couldn't believe it. The following morning, I went before the judge and was sentenced to go to the Women's prison until the Ontario police came to get me. I couldn't believe that this was happening to me.

The police handcuffed my hands and feet and put me in a van with other prisoners and we went to prison. I started to chat with the other prisoners in the van. I was still manic and chatty as this is one of the symptoms of mania. We finally arrived at the women's prison and they led me into the building. They removed our chains and handed us some clothing to wear, a pillow to sleep on, some utensils, soap and a toothbrush. I went up to my cell and met my roommate with a few other women smoking homemade cigarettes. My roommate was a meth addict and would go to the meth clinic for her dosages. However, she was a nice lady but spoke very little English. Being in prison wasn't too bad as I made friends very easily. This prison experience was better than the last one in 2013 where I put in the mental health ward. This time I was in the general public.

While there, I met a few people that stood out for me. There was the prison peer coordinator, an exotic dancer and a black woman who was a PSW. To keep busy, I started to plan out my businesses, one of which was to start to have parties in different cities with people wearing only Adidas. I thought it was a phenomenal idea. Others found it good as well. While there, I offered to pay the exotic dancer $500 to dance at one of my events in Toronto and Jamaica. She was excited about it. With the PSW, I told her that I would be opening up a hotel that she could work at once I was set free. She believed me because I believed me. Finally, with the peer coordinator, I told her that I would help find her a new lawyer and help her get out of jail because apparently she was in there for a crime she did not commit. Being the trusting person I was, I believed her story wholeheartedly. Though I was in prison, I still believed that this was just a minor setback and that I would be able to launch my businesses once I was released.

After six days of being in prison, the Ontario police finally arrived to Montreal by car to pick me up. I packed my stuff and went with the officers in handcuffs into the backseat of the car. The officers were very nice. They played really cool music and chatted with me. It was a long ride back home. We stopped once at an OPP station along the highway to stretch our legs and continued the journey to Oshawa. When I arrived in Oshawa, I went into the jail and waited till it was time to go to court. It was a lengthy process but finally, it was time for me to go to court and my mother and godmother were at the courthouse. I was released under the care of my mother, as she was a surety for me. I was truly thankful to be out of prison but in order to be released, I had to live with my mother for a minimum of one month so that she could monitor me take my medications. Though relieved, I was not happy to be at my mother's house. I wanted to be back so I could be close to my son. I was starting to miss him dearly.

Living with my mother was a bit difficult as I was so used to being alone. I felt as though I was under a microscope. However, I was simply happy to be out of prison. While at my mom's house, I decided to make a post on social media about my experience. I wrote the following on February 7, 2018,

> "Social media family, I need your prayers. I just came out of women's prison in Montreal for uttering threats while ill. I'm frustrated. I am remorseful and wish I could take it back but I can't. While ill, my son has been with his new godmother/babysitter. She has been a godsend. She has taken care of my baby as if it were her own. I miss my baby so much but I know that I need to be well first. While in prison for a few days, I met some genuine people who have been screwed over by the law. Please don't judge, I'm doing the best I can. Not all people who end up in jail belong there. I belonged in the hospital not jail. With that said,

that's where I'm taking myself to. I'm gonna check into CAMH to see why the meds aren't working for the Bipolar they say I have and to also get treated for my PTSD and GAD (Generalized Anxiety Disorder). I want to get to the root of my problems. I refuse to give up no matter how many times life hits me down. I'm a fighter! I shall overcome and THIS TOO SHALL PASS! Family and friends, keep me in prayers. I miss my son."

The post I made got 31 likes, 5 loves, 4 sad emoji's, 1 shocked emoji and 25 comments. Despite how many times I had failed, I was thankful to know that people were still praying for me. Once I made the post, I got my bag ready and went to CAMH to see if they would take me in. Unfortunately, they said they could not help me and that I should see my ACT team. With that advice, I contacted my ACT team and we talked about changing my medication. They decided that they would add Zyprexa to my dosage and would temporarily set me up with the West Metro ACT team while living with my mom. Though I was living at my mother's, I would still take the bus two hours to see my son at Margaret's house. Despite it being so far, I had to return back home to my mother's house after each visit. I simply hated being so far from my son but this was the consequence of my actions.

The month of me living with my mother finally ended and I was so happy to move back home and be near my son. With all the craziness, I had decided that I would not return back to fashion school that semester and would focus on getting my son back. While back home, I would visit my son at Margaret's as often as I could. However, it was not the same as having him in my house with me. In order to see him, I would have to schedule it with Margaret and would get to take him to church on some Sundays. At one point there was tension between Margaret and I but thankfully, we are in a good place now.

In order to get my son back in my care, I had to prove to Children's Aid that I could care for him independently by following specific steps. Gradually over the months, they would increase my visits and give me the chance to have him unsupervised in my home. However, over the months, I always had to have supervised visits with my son. This also included church. I could not go to church with him alone. In order to go to church, I had to have someone that was approved to carry me and watch me while in service. This approved person had to check in with my worker Leslie. This was heartbreaking. After months of following the rules, on July 20, 2018, my son was returned to my care on a Supervisory order of 6 months. What that meant was that for 6 months, weekly I had to meet with my worker at my home with my son. This was annoying but I was lucky to have a really great worker. She made the process very tolerable.

Due to the pregnancy and my medication, I had gained a lot of weight, over 80 lbs., and was desperate to lose the weight. For the first time ever, I had a large stomach and was quite heavy. I decided that I would join a gym and start losing the weight. I joined the Fit4Less location close to my home. Since I was used to making videos on social media, I thought that I would chronicle my journey day by day. So each day, I would walk 25 minutes to the gym, make a video there while working out for about an hour or more, and then walk back. I repeated this journey five days a week and was starting to lose the weight. I was feeling good about myself and at the same time I was inspiring others. Every Friday, I would weigh in. I called it #ResultsFriday. I was so consistent with this that the head office at Fit4Less noticed my videos and photos. They contacted me and asked if they could repost one of my videos. I was so excited and agreed. They posted my photo on their page and I got many likes. To date, I have lost almost 40 lbs. and the difference is noticeable. Going to the gym has really been good for my mental health. I was so glad I started.

It had been months since I had had a manic attack and I was doing really well. People were very proud of me. I was raising my son and doing a really great job. With this progress, the Pregnancy Care Centre invited me to an Alumni meeting where we discussed school, work and financial aid for school. At the end of the meeting, we showed the new website and a few of the videos of mothers sharing their stories on their new YouTube channel. They gave us the opportunity to share our story and I told them that I was interested. A month later, a meeting was scheduled for me to record my interview about mental health and pregnancy. The interview was originally 30 minutes but they edited it down to 10 minutes. When they finally posted it on their YouTube channel, I shared it with everyone on social media, WhatsApp and in my favorite group, the Black Moms Connection. After sharing it, I had received to date 290 views, which were the most views that any of their videos had received.

Considering how much time had elapsed since I had been sick, I started to think about my future and career. With my OSAP (student loans) being paid off, I now qualified for new loans for school. So, I struggled with the idea of what to study if I went to school. Centennial College was offering a new program called Addiction and Mental Health that I found very interesting. However, I strongly felt like I should finish what I started and study fashion. After thinking it through and speaking with people on my ACT team;

Harsha, Maisha, Lawrence and Geetha, I decided that I would finish my program in fashion.

However, I hadn't sewn anything in months. I did not feel the same drive and inspiration I once felt. Despite this, I pushed passed those feelings and went to the George Brown fashion office and told them that I was considering returning to school in September 2019. Considering how I left school earlier that year, I would need to speak to the coordinator to get permission to re-enter the program. They told me to email the coordinator and I did. However, I did not receive an email back. While waiting on the email, I started to feel that fashion wasn't for me. So, I changed my mind and decided that I would take the Addictions and Mental Health program.

I shared this news with the team and they responded positively as they knew I would make a great mental health worker. They believed I had a lot to offer the mental health industry. So, I decided to apply to the Centennial College in January 2019. This program was also offered at Durham College but I did not want to go to Durham College because it was too far. I wanted to be close to school and Centennial College was pretty close by. Once I applied I shared this with my ACT team and got the thumbs up. A few weeks had passed and then one morning as I was checking my email, on Friday February 1st, 2019, I received an email that I had been accepted into the program. I literally jumped off my bed and started jumping up and down, as this was amazing news. I immediately, screenshot the letter and posted it on my social media pages and my favorite group, the Black Moms Connection. The women in the Black Moms Connection were very excited for me, as they liked it 316 times with 42 congratulatory comments.

The following morning, I went to the CMHA office for my Friday visit and I was so excited to share my news. I shared it with my nurse Kate and she was very happy for me. Since I had recently met with another worker on the team, Wayne, once I was done talking to Kate, I asked if I could quickly give him a high five. He came out the office and I gave him a high five for getting in school. I then, sent my worker Maisha a text with the good news. She responded a few days later with excitement. Life was looking good for me.

   For years, I had struggled with finding a meaning for my life. I tried many different paths and businesses over the years, but I haven't felt as much peace as I did when I decided to enter the Addictions and Mental Health Worker program. I am so glad I decided on this path and I believe it will give all the pain and trials that I went through a meaning. I needed to know the purpose of my illness. Now, I know what that purpose was, so I want to share my story and give back. This is the year that I give back. This is the year that I give all of me for the cause.

www.ingramcontent.com/pod-product-compliance
Lightning Source LLC
Chambersburg PA
CBHW052249220526
45471CB00001B/256